THE HEALTHIEST YOU

THE HEALTHIEST YOU

Take Charge of Your Brain to
Take Charge of Your Life

Previously published as
The Program: The Brain-Smart Approach to the Healthiest You:
The Life-Changing 12-Week Method

KELLY TRAVER, M.D.

AND

BETTY KELLY SARGENT

ATRIA PAPERBACK

New York   London   Toronto   Sydney   New Delhi

This publication contains the opinions and ideas of the author. It is sold with the understanding that the author and publisher are not engaged in rendering health services in the book. The reader should consult his or her own medical and health providers as appropriate before adopting any of the suggestions in this book or drawing inferences from it.

The author and publisher specifically disclaim all responsibility for any liability, loss or risk, personal or otherwise, which is incurred as a consequence, directly or indirectly, of the use and application of any of the contents of this book.

ATRIA PAPERBACK

A Division of Simon & Schuster, Inc.
1230 Avenue of the Americas
New York, NY 10020

Copyright © 2009 by Kelly Traver, M.D., and Elizabeth Kelly Sargent

Previously published as *The Program: The Brain-Smart Approach to the Healthiest You*

First Atria Paperback edition December 2011

ATRIA PAPERBACK and colophon are trademarks of Simon & Schuster, Inc.

For information about special discounts for bulk purchases, please contact Simon & Schuster Special Sales at 1-866-506-1949 or business@simonandschuster.com.

The Simon & Schuster Speakers Bureau can bring authors to your live event. For more information or to book an event, contact the Simon & Schuster Speakers Bureau at 1-866-248-3049 or visit our website at www.simonspeakers.com.

Designed by Joel Avirom and Jason Snyder
Illustrations by Paul Martini

Manufactured in the United States of America

10 9 8 7 6 5 4 3 2 1

The Library of Congress cataloged the hardcover edition as follows:
Traver, Kelly.
    The program : the brain-smart approach to the healthiest you :
    the life-changing 12-week method / by Kelly Traver and
    Betty Kelly Sargent. —1st. ed.
    p. cm.
    Includes index.
    1. Clinical health psychology. 2. Health behavior. 3. Neuropsychology. I. Sargent,
Betty Kelly. II. Title.
    R726.7.T73 2009
    613—dc22   2009018253

ISBN 978-1-4391-0998-4
ISBN 978-1-4391-0999-1 (pbk)
ISBN 978-1-4391-4968-3 (ebook)

To my beautiful family
for their love, support, and encouragement.
Thank you for always believing in me.
—KELLY TRAVER, M.D.

For Elizabeth Lee Kelly, my heroine,
and for John, James, Izabela, and Xavier.
—BETTY KELLY SARGENT

CONTENTS

INTRODUCTION

WHEN I OPENED MY INTERNAL MEDICINE PRACTICE at Menlo Medical Clinic in Menlo Park, California, in 1993, I couldn't have been happier. Medicine gave me everything I wanted in a job: It was intellectually challenging, required constant learning, and, best of all, I got to work with people and develop relationships that would last for years. With accomplished colleagues and an amazing group of patients, I couldn't have designed a better job for myself.

But as time went on, I began to notice a disturbing trend. I saw more and more people who were struggling to stay healthy. Increasingly, people were finding it harder to fit exercise into their lives, to maintain their weight, and to manage stress. It wasn't that people weren't trying, but the American way of life, for many people, had become a roadblock to the pursuit of health. What's more, the U.S. health care system seemed geared to treating illness, not to promoting health effectively.

As medical journals' headlines featured skyrocketing cases of diabetes and obesity, it was announced that life expectancy in the United States had fallen to last place among all of the developed countries in the world. This is when I decided I wanted to come up with a better way of practicing medicine. How could the United States be spending more money on health than any other country on the planet and have such poor results?

In almost any analysis of health trends, the data show that lifestyle behavior accounts for 50 percent of one's health. Lifestyle also accounts for 50 percent of the total cost of health care and 50 percent of the total causes of death. Genetics influence 20 percent, environment 20 percent, and access to quality health care 10 percent. It seemed clear to me that to improve health, we had to focus more on helping people improve their lifestyle behavior.

Surely, I thought, we can learn to use our brains better to help us live a healthy life. I have always been fascinated with the human brain. During medical school, I worked as a teaching assistant at Stanford in a neuroanatomy lab, dissecting human cadaver brains and teaching medical students about the brain's function. But that was twenty years ago, in the late 1980s; the past ten years of neuroscience research have exploded with new information on how the brain works. I became convinced that the most effective healthy living program would need to incorporate the past decade of brain research into its design. I was also determined to build my new method, The Program, on solid, evidence-based studies, free from gimmicks and fads, and to teach people how everything in their health was interconnected.

So in January 2005 I sent a letter to my patients asking them if they wanted to participate in a pilot program in which I hoped to develop the ultimate toolbox for healthy living. I could take only fifty patients, and the cost of The Program wouldn't be covered by health insurance, so I wasn't sure how much of a response I would get. By noon of the first day, thirty people had called to say they wanted to join, and by day two we had our fifty volunteers and had to close the doors. I was amazed by how many people wanted to take on this challenge and learn more about their health and what they could do to optimize it.

This first group ranged in age from 20 to 81 years and was made up of an equal number of men and women. Their goals were varied. Many people wanted to lose weight, but others were interested in managing their diabetes, cholesterol, and blood pressure. Some were worried about the enormous amount of stress they felt in their lives or were experiencing depression or anxiety. Some were quite healthy but just wanted to learn more to keep their healthy lifestyle going.

The results of this first pilot study were truly encouraging. The participants were able to make enormous strides, which have, in most cases, been maintained for years. Here is a summary of the remarkable health results they achieved.

- Of those who were overweight, there was on average:

  - A 15% reduction in body fat

  - A 19-pound weight loss

  - A 7.5% reduction in BMI

- Of those who were diabetic or prediabetic:

  - 80% achieved reduction of their blood sugar level

  - 60% achieved normalization of their blood sugar level

- Of those who had high blood pressure:

  - 98% achieved reduction of their blood pressure

  - 87% achieved normalization of their blood pressure

- Of those with high cholesterol:

  - 14% achieved reduction of their LDL cholesterol level

  - 17% achieved elevation of their HDL cholesterol level

- 80% of smokers achieved tobacco cessation.

- The vast majority of patients also experienced better sleep, higher energy levels, and improved mood.

After this positive experience, I decided to open a health center dedicated to helping people live proactively to stay healthy. I wanted to experiment with different models to find a program that would be effective yet affordable and reach out to the largest number of people possible. As I designed different programs, more and more people enrolled. Doctors referred patients to the new center, and many people came in self-referred; they had heard about The Program from past participants.

Within the first year I was also asked to bring the program on site to the Google headquarters in Mountain View, California. Google was forward-thinking and proactive about taking care of its employees. Ultimately, The Program was offered to all Google employees in the United States. Over time, other corporations came to us, as did community centers, medical clinics, and athletic centers. Patients, doctors, and employers alike saw the need for a more take-charge approach to health.

After the first year we began to get calls from people from all over the country asking if they could participate in the program. At first we pieced together a way to deliver the information and work with individuals one-on-one by telephone or by e-mail, but it was clear that we needed to develop a better way to deliver The Program to anyone anywhere. In 2007 we launched The Program online and offered two different ways of participating. The first involved working with a personal coach either online or by phone, while learning the information through short videos. The second method supplied the participant with all the information and tools online but taught that person how to be his or her own best coach.

In 2007 Stanford University heard about The Program and undertook a formal research study involving a number of sites around the nation. The study looked at the twelve-week online program, which included e-mail and phone coaching. Its results confirmed significant progress by participants in the areas of weight loss, cholesterol level, and blood pressure reduction. Stanford University now offers The Program to all its employees.

In 2008 we began to work with the Centers for Disease Control and Prevention (CDC) and a newly created nonprofit organization called the Alliance to Make U.S. Healthiest. In 2009, we also began working with the Healthy People Consortium and Healthy 2020 with the Human Health Services Department. Today, many large and small corporate and government groups are coming together to help promote healthful behavior all across the country. A national movement has begun. We have committed The Program to this effort.

This movement is happening everywhere, and I encourage you to be part of it. As you get started with The Program, I encourage you to form a group of friends to work with. Feel free to consult our website at www.theprogrambook .com as you go forward. You will find useful videos, tips, downloadable material, incentives, and other speacial features to help you achieve your goals. Take it one step at a time, and remember: You can, without question, learn to be in the driver's seat of your own health.

Kelly Traver, M.D.

April 2009

PART I | YOUR BEAUTIFUL BRAIN

> Life is 10 percent what happens to you
> and 90 percent how you react.
> —CHARLES SWINDOLL

IT IS RARE TO FIND SOMEONE who doesn't want to live a happy, healthy life. Who doesn't want health? But *wanting* to live healthfully is one thing; *doing it* is quite another. Change can be a tricky process, so the more you know about it, the better. I have worked with thousands of patients, and what I see time and again is that people have a definite advantage when they understand how interconnected everything in their body is when it comes to health and how their brain works when it comes to change.

If you want to be as healthy as you can, you need to understand how everything affects everything else in the health department. It is not just about the food you eat or the exercise you do, although these two behaviors are extremely important. It is also about how you sleep, how you think, how you handle stress, and how you feel about the life you are living.

I'm convinced that the reason so many people on The Program have had such astonishing success is that they have learned how to appreciate and take advantage of the remarkable interconnections among their body, brain, and lifestyle. Equally important, they have learned how their brain works so that they can get it to cooperate with them when it comes to making positive, healthful changes.

I have two goals for you as you read this book. The first is to help you understand how amazingly interconnected everything in your health is. If you want to get healthier, you need to focus on all aspects of your lifestyle. The second is to teach you about your brain and how it operates reflexively. For example, one of the things it reacts against, reflexively, is change. I will explain why this happens and show you how to coax your brain into accepting change by introducing new behaviors *gradually*.

In the past decade, amazing groundbreaking research has revolutionized our understanding of the human brain. With all this new information we can, for the first time, learn to harness our brainpower so that it will work for us instead of against us, and we can do so in sophisticated ways that we never understood before. I'm going to tell you all about this research so you can put this new information into action as you set out to change your life for the better. In fact, I intend to teach you how to get your brain to be your best friend.

There are twelve major themes that explain the brain and its behavior, and I'll be discussing them all below. As you read through this book, you will see that all of these principles are carefully woven into The Program. I believe that the combination of understanding the material, and using it in a way that works with the brain's natural tendencies, is the secret of The Program's success and will be the secret of your success, too.

Although you may be tempted to skip ahead to part II, I encourage you to read through this section on how your brain works. Knowledge is power, and your ability to understand the way your brain operates can give you a definite edge in your efforts to live healthy. If, however, you choose to skip ahead to part II, know that there will be opportunities to go back and learn the brain material. For example, I will highlight one brain principle at the end of each week and list real-life examples of how past participants have put this information into action. I have also summarized all of the brain principles and listed concrete examples of how to use them.

The real trick in making any change is simply to get your brain to cooperate with you. I can assure you that your brain is perfectly capable of making all of the changes necessary to lead a healthy, happy life.

1. YOUR ADAPTABLE BRAIN

Your brain is incredibly adaptable and fully capable of change and, in fact, changes throughout your life. This first brain-behavior principle cannot be overstated. We are all capable of change. We can improve on what we are good at and eventually learn to do some of the things we thought were impossible. *As we learn new material and practice new behavior, changes occur both functionally and structurally within our brains.* This is quite remarkable when you think about it: we can actually physically restructure our brains based on the information we give it and the things we do.

The ever-changing nature of the brain is evident long before birth. A developing human embryo generates 250,000 neurons (nerve cells) *per minute.* Just

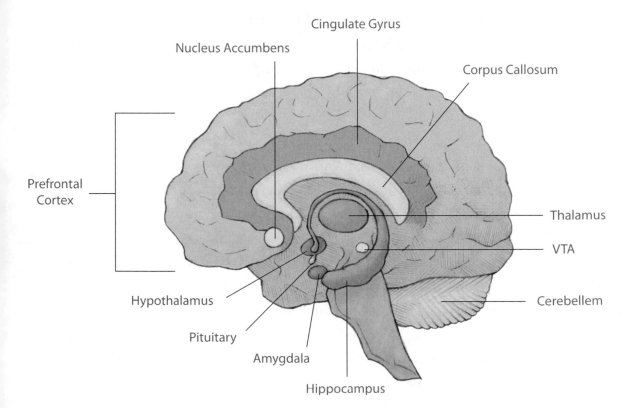

before birth, there is a sudden regression of neurons as the system "fine-tunes," causing as many as 70 percent of neurons to die in some areas of the brain. Even so, with all this loss, the adult human brain contains one hundred billion neurons, each neuron connecting to other neurons, resulting in more than one hundred trillion nerve-to-nerve connections. Now that's a lot of neurons!

As a baby grows, developmental milestones are reached. For example, the baby starts to walk and talk and recognize his mommy and daddy. These milestones become possible only as the infant's nerve system develops. The brain doesn't finish the maturation process until you are well into adulthood. It is not until one's midtwenties that the **frontal cortex** (the area of rational thought and one's impulse control) finally completes maturation. Hmmm . . . now, that explains a few things.

But the changes that occur in the brain don't stop here. We used to think that we were born with a finite number of nerve cells that slowly regressed and died throughout our lifetime. Wrong. A full decade of research has demonstrated conclusively that this is false. In addition to the lifelong formation of new nerve cell connections within the brain, some areas of the brain, such as the **hippocampus** (the memory center), retain the ability to form new neurons, even late in life. So in fact you can teach old dogs new tricks!

Additional factors also influence how the brain develops and changes. Depression and stress stimulate the production of chemicals such as cortisol that can damage and sometimes even kill neurons. In severe cases, the toxic, high levels of cortisol actually shrink the hippocampus and frontal cortex. You can see this with your own eyes in the fMRI images of some brains.

Exercise and mental stimulation, on the other hand, promote the production of chemicals such as brain-derived neurotrophic growth factor (BDNF) that encourage new growth. Sometimes you can even see these changes with the naked eye when looking at imaging studies. In a professional pianist or violinist, for example, the region of the brain that corresponds to finger movement grows to occupy a much larger area. In contrast, if you take one eye of a rat and seal it shut, the visual cortex of its brain (which processes visual information) shrinks. Your brain is like a muscle: use it or lose it.

An extreme example of the remarkable adaptive capacity of the brain has been seen in research done over the last few years in many different centers around the United States. In this research undifferentiated human nerve cells are injected into the brains of brain-damaged rats. These undifferentiated cells miraculously migrate from the ventricles of the inner brain right over to the damaged areas of the rat's brain. They then differentiate, or turn themselves into the correct types of nerve cells and supporting cells that naturally belong in these areas of the brain. Finally they integrate into the surrounding tissue. Absolutely amazing!

In 2008 at the University of California at Irvine, Frank LaFerla and his colleagues showed how injected neural stem cells can actually reverse memory loss in mice. By genetic manipulation, these scientists produced a group of mice with preprogrammed nerve cell death in their hippocampus so that these mice demonstrated significant memory loss. The scientists then injected neural stem cells that migrated to the damaged hippocampus, forming many new nerve connections.

Only 5 percent of the injected stem cells actually survived, but they produced growth factors that ultimately induced the proliferation of new nerve-to-nerve connections. After the transplantation, the impaired mice could perform just as well as the healthy mice!

More studies are under way to look at how Parkinson's disease, Alzheimer's dementia, and other neurological diseases might benefit from this type of therapy. Scientists are particularly interested in looking at how injection of these growth factors might stimulate nerve growth without requiring the actual injection of stem cells. This research truly demonstrates how remarkably resilient the human brain is and what great potential it has for change.

In fact, new research shows the ability to coax the fibroblast cells of the skin to transform into undifferentiated cells that can then be transplanted into any tissue of the body, where it then develops into new, specialized cells for that particular tissue. This could revolutionize the treatment of diseases ranging from Alzheimer's dementia to heart failure.

CONCLUSION: *Your brain is capable of substantial change. At any age, you can learn, you can grow, and you can improve your skills for living a healthier and happier life.*

2. YOUR RESISTANT BRAIN

Although your brain can change, it usually won't do so without putting up a bit of a fight. That's because it is set up to resist change, especially sudden change. Your brain operates under the same principle as your body: *homeostasis.* Just as your body's physiology works to keep parameters such as calcium, blood sugar, and weight stable, so your brain works hard to continue whatever behavior has become the norm. It seems to say, "Okay, I got you here with this behavior and you're still alive, so just keep on doing what you've been doing and everything will be fine." Your **hypothalamus,** in the center of your brain, is the master controller of homeostasis. The hypothalamus controls things like hunger, thirst, and body temperature. It also determines whether your stress response fires and whether reproductive hormones are released. The list of duties performed by your hypothalamus is long. All of the other parts of the brain, especially your emotional **limbic system,** fight to influence the hypothalamus.

Too rapid a change is interpreted as a stressful event by most brains. Your brain will automatically resist a sudden change in your behavior or routine, and just knowing this can be a big help when you are trying to switch from a not-so-healthful behavior to a healthful one. Studies using functional MRI scans of the brain have evaluated patients who were asked to make a change. If a patient is asked to make a big change, the scan shows activation of the **amygdala** (a-MIG-

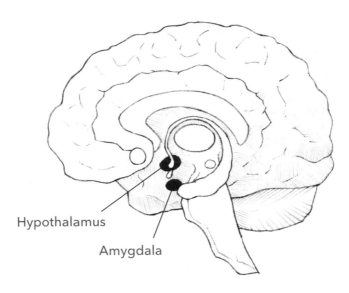

Hypothalamus

Amygdala

duh-luh), the seat of the stress response. But if the subject is asked to make a small change, the amygdala remains quiet. People who are ultimately successful in initiating and maintaining major behavioral change usually do it through gradual, step-by-step changes. That's how The Program works and, actually, why it works so well. I know it isn't always easy to wait for results that take place gradually. People usually want instant gratification, but for most of us this just isn't realistic. We need to accept the fact that most people's brains are not well set up to handle rapid change. For the majority of us, slow and steady change is actually the quickest road to long-lasting results.

If you feel your motivation beginning to slip, it is probably because your brain is saying "Oh no, you don't! I sense a change here, and I'm not going to let that happen." This can leave you feeling frustrated and confused. How, you ask yourself, can you so desperately want to make a change one day but then come up with a thousand reasons not to the next? When this happens, remind yourself that this is simply an example of your brain working against you—doing what it thinks it has to do to protect you. You can outsmart it, though. Your brain will start to feel more comfortable with your new actions once you have repeated the new behavior many times, so start repeating the new action over and over again.

Another way to help your brain accept change is to work within a structure. Your brain is very rule-based, so it generally feels more comfortable when the rules are clearly defined. It takes less energy for your brain when you have a clear set of rules to guide it than when you have to make new decisions all along the way. The trick with structure, though, is that if you want to create lasting behavior change, you need to learn how to perform a behavior in all sorts of situations that may be outside the structure you are following. I know this sounds a little complicated, but it's really not. Let's look at the example of a weight loss plan that tells you exactly what to eat.

You may be very successful while you are on the diet because you don't need to make any decisions about what to eat, but after you have lost the weight you have no idea how to eat in a healthful way on your own. The diet didn't teach you that. Certainly, structure can be very helpful in the beginning, but pay attention to *the process within the structure.* The process (in this case the original diet) should show you how to create your own rules--rules that you can live with forever. This is what The Program is designed to do.

As you can see, it is not always easy to change the way you behave, but the good news is that you *can* do it. We know that if you practice a new behavior over and over for a long enough period of time, your brain will eventually decide that this new behavior is the one that needs to be protected and continued. The key words here are "over and over." You need to repeat the new behavior for long enough to cement it permanently into your brain and therefore into your life.

CONCLUSION: *Although your brain can change, it is generally set up to resist change, especially sudden change. People who are ultimately successful in initiating and maintaining major behavioral changes usually make the changes gradually, one step at a time.*

3. YOUR RATIONAL BRAIN

The **frontal cortex** of your brain is the highly developed area that allows for problem solving. This is where sophisticated levels of thought processing occur and where information is processed so that you can understand it. Knowing why you do what you do and having an appreciation for the potential consequences of your actions can help shape your behavior.

It is also the center of impulse control. It promotes delayed gratification and helps you behave within the social mores of society. It can help you "do the more difficult thing" when other parts of your brain are calling for you to do something else. It allows you to check and balance yourself so that you don't act impulsively with every temptation that comes your way. As I've mentioned before, this part of the brain has not fully finished developing until an adult's midtwenties, and this plays a role in the high-risk behavior sometimes seen in teenagers.

What happens if the frontal cortex is destroyed? In the 1850s, a famous accident occurred. A young man named Phineas Gage was working as a foreman on a railroad. He was a well-mannered, hardworking young man, but one day there was a dynamite explosion and a huge piece of metal flew into his skull, blowing right through the frontal cortex of his brain. He was thrown to the ground, but, according to the story, he never lost consciousness. He picked himself up and walked a mile to get to the nearest doctor. After the accident, Phineas Gage was largely unaffected in his ability to think and perform tasks. With his damaged frontal cortex, though, he was no longer able to control his impulses or make rational, thoughtful decisions. He started drinking, gambling, and using profanity. He could no longer hold down a job. Everyone who knew him felt he had become an entirely different person after the accident. In clinical medicine today, we see this type of behavior in certain neurological conditions such as frontotemporal dementia, in which the frontal lobe shrinks over time.

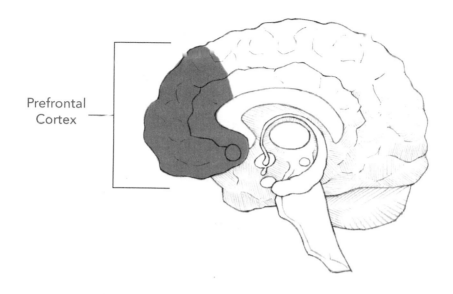

Prefrontal
Cortex

The frontal cortex is specifically developed for problem solving. It is often called the chief executive officer, or CEO, of the brain. The left hemisphere specializes in linear, analytical problem solving, while the right hemisphere is more involved in visual or spatial problem solving. The left hemisphere tends to look at data in discrete chunks, whereas the right tends to view the data as a whole. Some people problem-solve with a more left-brain-dominant, linear, logical, "if A, then B" type of thinking. Other people are more right-brain-dominant and create more nonlinear solutions. No one, of course, works purely from one side of the brain or the other, because both sides of the brain are connected to the **corpus callosum,** a thick highway of nerve bundles that allows the two sides to communicate with each other. In problem solving, especially as it relates to healthy behavior, there is almost never only one answer for how to get from A to B. Ultimately, success is determined not so much by how much willpower you can muster when you face challenges; it is more about how well you can strategize around these challenges. You need to learn how to confront challenges in a way that will best work for you as an individual.

Although rational intellectual thought does play a role in behavior, it is important to understand that much of rational decision making does not occur without emotional input; in fact, there is a very tight connection between the rational and emotional areas of the brain. The higher cognitive areas of the frontal cortex receive massive input from the emotional **limbic system** that sits in the deeper brain. The limbic system is far older evolutionarily than the much more recently developed cognitive frontal cortex. Because of this interconnection, like it or not, your behavior is greatly influenced by your emotions.

Here is an example of how emotional input influences rational thought. In 2001, at Princeton's Center for Brain, Mind and Behavior, the results of a fascinating study were published. In this study functional brain MRI scans were performed on subjects asked to answer the "runaway trolley" question. In this classic philosophical dilemma, a trolley is headed toward five people. If the trolley continues, it will kill all five people, but if a lever is pulled, the trolley will switch to an alternative track with only one person standing on it. The subject is asked if he or she will pull the lever.

Most people say they will pull the lever in order to sacrifice one person to save five. As the subject thinks about the question, the functional MRI scan shows activation within the frontal cortex of rational thought. There is only a little input from the emotional limbic system. Now, if the scenario is changed and the subject is told that in order to save the five people he or she will have to physically push one person in front of the trolley rather than simply pull a lever, all of a sudden the limbic system springs into action; there is a tremendous amount of cross talk from the emotional center to the frontal cortex. In this exercise, most people refuse to save five people by sacrificing one. Both exercises involve taking an action to save five lives by sacrificing one, but the emotional context is clearly different in the second situation. This changes the thought processing in the brain, and a flurry of emotional input reverses the original decision.

The French philosopher René Descartes (1596–1650) was a big champion of the concept called "dualism." According to this theory, the human mind and body are completely separate entities. With time, it has become very clear there is no such separation. In the 1992 book, *Descartes' Error,* the University of Iowa neurologist Antonio Damasio wrote about Elliot, a young man who required surgery for a brain tumor. The surgery required severing the pathways that connected his frontal and limbic regions. After the surgery his frontal cortex could no longer get input from the emotional limbic center. Elliot could no longer feel any emotion. Without the frontal cortex, he had no framework in which to set the emotional input from the limbic system. Also, to everyone's surprise, he could no longer make a decision. He could intelligently weigh the advantages and disadvantages of various solutions to a problem, but he could not actually make a decision. Making decisions often requires input from the emotional limbic center, as we saw in the runaway trolley experiment. The frontal cortex does not operate in isolation. In fact, there are more connections traveling to the frontal cortex from the emotional limbic system than from anywhere else in the brain.

Because the "intellectual" and "emotional" centers are so tightly connected, you cannot rely purely on willpower (governed by the intellectual part of your brain) when you want to make a change. None of us is exclusively a creature of rational thought. Our emotions have a lot to do with our actions. The great news in all of this is that *we are capable of altering both cognitive and emotional input.* We can even use the connections between the intellectual and emotional brains to our advantage by learning to enhance positive emotions while diminishing the negative ones. By understanding both how to use your emotional brain to influence your rational brain and how to use your rational brain to influence your emotional brain, you can have a big impact on changing your behavior.

One way of doing this is to reframe your emotions through conscious thought. For example, when you are stressed, your sympathetic nervous system increases your heart rate and blood pressure, and stress chemicals are released. Your brain can interpret these physiologic changes in two completely different ways. In one scenario, you feel immense dread because it is the middle of the night, you are hearing noises downstairs and, you interpret this to mean that someone must be breaking into your house. In another scenario, you experience exactly the same stress physiology but you are on a roller coaster, scared to death yet having the time of your life. In other words, your cerebral cortex frames all incoming information within a certain context.

Mary had traveled on planes her whole life without fear until one day, shortly after her first baby was born, she developed a fear of flying. She was fine getting onto a plane but would panic whenever the plane experienced turbulence. It was a terrible feeling, and she couldn't shake it by trying to talk herself through it logically. So she decided that whenever the plane started shaking she would imagine she was in a James Bond car racing around in some kind of dramatic car chase, or she'd imagine she was having fun on a roller coaster. It might sound silly, but it worked. She made it through hours of turbulence during an extremely bumpy flight from Nashville to San Francisco where the flight attendants were not even allowed to get out of their seats. She and her daughter (who played "roller coaster" with her) even laughed and had some good moments together on that flight. Ultimately, Mary overcame her fear, although she still uses this strategy whenever a plane ride becomes especially turbulent.

Your brain is also playful and creative. This is often overlooked when we discuss problem solving or cognitive thought. Your brain loves to play. It thrives on riddles and questions. As you confront problems along the way, try to help your brain think of answers by posing your challenges as questions. For example, Joan, a 39-year-old mother of two and part-time medical assistant, had always assumed she was "lazy" because she never found the time to exercise. But when she really began to ask herself why she never found the time, she realized that she truly did have a lot on her plate and also felt "selfish" taking time for herself when she exercised. She knew that exercise was valid, important, and worthwhile in its own right, but she still veered away from it because she felt it was "unproductive time." So she solved her problem in a creative way. She wanted to learn how to speak Spanish for her work as a medical assistant. She decided to teach herself Spanish; she made flash cards and quizzed herself while walking on her home treadmill. This made the time pass quickly for her, and she felt good about the time she was exercising because she felt she was being productive. Your brain can be very creative when it comes to problem solving

CONCLUSION: *Human beings are highly intellectual and creative creatures. Your brain is well designed for problem solving. Keep this in mind, and use it to your advantage when you run into challenges with healthful living.*

4. YOUR EMOTIONAL BRAIN

In addition to their role in rational decision making, emotions have a profound impact on how we experience life. Fortunately, we can learn to enhance our positive emotions and play down the negative ones that get in our way—a skill that can help us more than any other when it comes to making positive, long-lasting changes in the way we live.

Your emotions are housed in your limbic system, an anatomic structure in the core of your brain. Within the limbic system, the amygdala plays a leading role. The amygdala is the seat of the stress response and fires whenever it senses danger, activating the infamous "fight-or-flight" response. As you now know, activity within the limbic system affects the activity within your frontal cortex.

When you are stressed, for example, your frontal cortex receives less blood flow and is therefore less able to engage in higher levels of thinking. When you experience the stress response, your brain and body are set up for "fight or flight." This gives you quicker reflexes and heightened senses, but it is not an optimal setting for complex problem solving. All your brain—and therefore your body— cares about in this situation is being able to fight or run to safety.

Stress inflicted on animals, including humans, causes a withering of nerve cells. Recently, it has been shown in rats that stress can kill nerve cells. In 2007 Daniel Peterson and his colleagues at Rosalind Franklin University of Medicine

THE LIMBIC SYSTEM

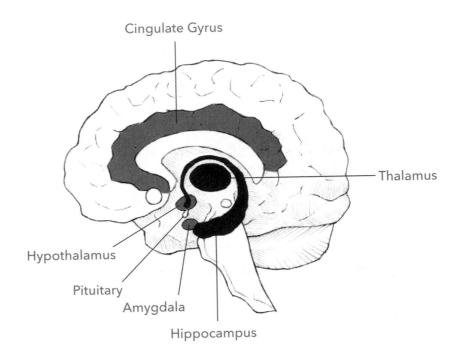

Cingulate Gyrus

Thalamus

Hypothalamus

Pituitary

Amygdala

Hippocampus

and Science demonstrated that when a young adult rat was introduced into a cage with two older rats who behaved aggressively, not only did the stress level in the new rat increase to six times normal, *two thirds* of the newly generated nerve cells in its hippocampus were destroyed!

Your brain also reacts to the microenvironment of neurotransmitters and hormones with which it has direct contact. Hippocampal nerve cells are rich in **cortisol receptors,** so the hippocampus is a prime target in both stress and depression. When you are stressed or depressed, your cortisol levels run high. In severe, untreated depression and severe prolonged stress, the hippocampus can actually be seen to visibly shrink on MRI imaging scans, as I've mentioned. Fortunately, in most but not all cases, once the stress is removed or the depression is treated, the nerve cells recover.

In a 2006 study at the Johns Hopkins University School of Medicine, rats given the antidepressant medication Prozac grew new nerve fibers in mood-critical areas of the brain. Although it had previously been known that Prozac and other similar antidepressants treated depression by increasing serotonin levels, this study was the first to report *anatomic changes* within the brain in response to an antidepressant. Exercise has actually been shown to do the very same thing, and in a 1999 Duke University study, exercise was shown to be more effective in the long term in reversing the effects of depression than was medication with antidepressants.

You can also learn how to turn off the stress response through deep breathing, meditation, or even mental imagery. You will learn more about this later in The Program, but for now I want you to know that you have a lot more control over what goes on in your brain and body than you probably think.

We often set goals and make decisions based on our feelings about these goals. This is not necessarily bad unless we have allowed too much negative emotion to impair our decision making. Negative emotion can simply overwhelm the decision-making process. You want to be able to direct your brain in a way that works *for* you and not *against* you. This is one of the most important skills you can learn in life.

You can start to manipulate your mood by engaging in activities that cause feel-good chemicals to be released. We'll talk more about this later in The Program, but for now just know that brain chemicals that go along with positive emotions are released through all sorts of pleasurable activities such as listening to music, watching a gorgeous sunset, reading, or playing soccer with your kids. Doing the things you enjoy stimulates your pleasure centers and reward systems. Sometimes just the anticipation of doing something you love can stimulate these pleasure centers. Learning how to enhance positive emotions and dampen negative ones can help decision making because the rational and emotional centers of the brain are inextricably intertwined. Your mind and body (and therefore your health) are also inextricably connected. To be in the driver's seat of your health means you must learn to be in the driver's seat of your brain.

Also, understand that not all stress is bad. Stress can actually be good in small doses. Performance goes up during brief periods of stress but down if the stress is chronic. You can learn better during short pulses of stress. You can also grow emotionally stronger from stress—a process referred to as *stress inoculation.* The key here is that the stress must be short term and you need to feel that you have some control over its outcome.

CONCLUSION: *The rational and emotional centers of your brain are tightly inter-connected. You can learn how to have a positive influence on your mood and modify your stress levels through well-defined strategies that can ultimately improve your ability to be healthy and happy.*

5. YOUR LEARNING BRAIN

One of the most remarkable aspects of the human mind is its tremendous capacity to learn. We are all different when it comes to how we learn best. Some of us prefer reading information, others prefer hearing it; some learn best by seeing graphic representations of information, others by interacting with the material. For most of us, the more methods we use while learning and the more senses we engage, the better we learn.

How do people learn? Learning involves a change in both the function and the structure of brain cells. When you learn something new, the ion channels of the nerve cell's membranes open up more easily to pass the resulting electrical message more quickly to the neuron next door. The better you have learned something, the more easily the message is relayed and the more easily the behavior is translated into action. This process works best with numerous, spaced-out repetitions; but not too many repetitions within a short time period. Yes, you've heard it before: practice *does* make perfect. The cardinal rule in learning anything, whether it is the multiplication tables or a new tennis serve, is that you

MEMORY CENTER

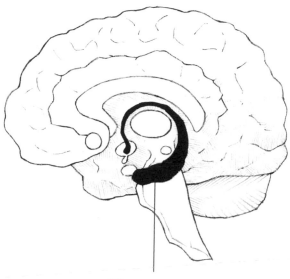

Hippocampus

need to *repeat the learning activity or behavior* over a period of time. Scientists call this long-term potentiation. I call it learning, but the important words in the scientific version are "long-term." This means that the effects of learning last a long time. In other words, after we have practiced a behavior over and over, it becomes easier. We don't have to work at it as hard. It becomes second nature. It becomes a habit.

In 2000 Dr. Eric Kandel of Columbia University won the Nobel Prize for his work on memory. He discovered that if nerve cells are stimulated repetitively, a gene is activated that prompts the production of a protein called cAMP response element binding (CREB), and this protein physically cements the changes in the brain. The existing synapses are tightened, and new synapses are created. As neuroscientists are fond of saying, "Neurons that fire together, wire together."

Right now there is active research to try to find and produce a drug that will elevate the CREB protein in the brain to enhance memory. This drug could be helpful in treating diseases in which memory is impaired, such as Alzheimer's dementia. Most people, however, don't need a drug to enhance their long-term memory. They just need to practice the learning behavior over and over again.

The structures of the brain responsible for long-term memory are the **hippocampus** and **cerebral cortex.** The hippocampus is necessary for learning new information; it is the initiator of memory, slowly transferring information into the cerebral cortex over many years. The hippocampus is one of the most severely affected structures in Alzheimer's dementia. The importance of the hippocampus was first noted in the 1950s through a patient referred to in the literature as H.M. H.M. suffered from seizures that originated in the hippocampus of both temporal lobes. His seizures occurred several times a day, were profoundly debilitating, and failed to respond to medication. In a desperate attempt to control the seizures, H.M.'s temporal lobes were surgically removed. The seizures did indeed decrease after the surgery, but the horrible side effect of the surgery was that H.M. could no longer remember anything for longer than thirty seconds. He did retain some long-term memory (since long-term memory is stored in both the hippocampus and cerebral cortex), but the loss of both his hippocampi prevented any new learning whatsoever. H.M. is still alive, but he requires twenty-four-hour care because he is so completely unable to learn and remember any new information.

We have recently discovered that the genders often differ in the way they learn and process information. In general, women tend to be stronger in both verbal and written communication and have particularly strong memories for faces, names, and events. Men tend to be more dominant in spatial skills, those used in building structures or navigating. Certainly, the culture in which one is raised can magnify these differences, but differences in the male and female brains exist even before birth.

You learn best when you find a topic interesting, important, and most of all relevant to your life. Information is retained best when seen in pictures or graphs, not just in text; your brain also remembers more when information is presented with color and motion. Finally, when information elicits strong emotions, good or bad, you are more likely to remember it.

The context in which you learn makes a difference, too. If you skip sleep, you lose out on the opportunity to consolidate what you have learned. This process is called memory consolidation, and it occurs as you sleep. Studies have consistently showed that those who try to memorize information do far better when they "sleep on it" than when they are sleep-deprived. During sleep, your brain is active, with neural networks firing repeatedly; this repetitive firing turns on genes and produces proteins that ultimately promote the formation of long-term modifications between the nerve-to-nerve connections. You also solve problems when you sleep as shown by a recent research study at Harvard Medical School and McGill University. Students in this study were given puzzle problems too difficult to figure out right away. Both groups were retested twelve hours later. The group that had been allowed to sleep was clearly able to outperform the group that had not slept. Sleeping can let the brain see a problem from a different perspective, making it easier to solve. Try it: the next time you are struggling with a problem, "sleep on it" and see if it makes a difference.

Being sick or stressed makes it harder to learn. When you are sick, your immune system produces chemicals called interleukins. These chemicals interfere with your brain's ability to store information. Chronic stress inhibits learning because it reduces neural activity in the higher cognitive centers. Short bursts of stress, however, such as when you have a last-minute deadline, can facilitate learning.

Learning is also best facilitated when your blood sugar level remains stable. The brain is very metabolically expensive; it uses a lot of sugar to function, especially when multitasking. Although the brain makes up only 2 percent of the total body mass, it uses 20 percent of your blood sugar supply. Eating regular meals that sustain an even blood sugar level (avoiding rapid rises and falls) helps the brain to think more efficiently. Finally, too much alcohol inhibits both learning and memory consolidation.

It is also important to remember that we learn from our mistakes. In 2007 a study at the University of Exeter in England showed that when students were presented with images that had previously led them into making a mistake, a warning signal flashed in their brains within a fraction of a second of seeing the image. What this shows us is that it's okay to make mistakes and "fail" because it enables your brain to learn and be that much more prepared the next time you are faced with the same problem. In fact, almost all people who ultimately succeed in giving up smoking or losing weight have had many attempts and failures before they actually succeed.

The brain has certain tricks it relies on for memory. We often teach these tricks to people who are trying to improve their memory. One memory trick is to compartmentalize information, to toss it into categories. This helps to keep information organized and allows easy recall, which helps us remember it, but sometimes this trick backfires, because it is not always clear which category a piece of information should be placed in. Information is often a continuation along a spectrum, and compartmentalizing it can create artificial boundaries. Things are frequently not black or white. They are usually some shade of gray, but that's not how we remember them. Having an all-or-nothing, black-and-white way of looking at everything can work against you. For example, you may think of yourself as "on" a diet or "off" a diet. If you are not exercising like crazy, you may decide you might as well not do any exercise at all. In matters of health, I like the 80/20 rule: If you follow healthy guidelines 80 percent of the time, you are likely to be healthy. In fact, this is worth repeating: you don't have to do everything perfectly to be healthy.

CONCLUSION: *Your brain has a tremendous capacity to learn. Enhance factors that optimize learning, such as getting enough sleep and reducing stress, and don't be afraid to make mistakes and stumble along the way. That's how we all learn. Your brain also remembers through repetition. Practice whatever behavior you are trying to adopt over and over. And remember, you don't have to do everything perfectly. Follow the 80/20 rule.*

6. YOUR MOTIVATED BRAIN

In the past decade, we have learned so much about motivation. Interestingly, the chemical that drives motivation is also linked to addiction. The brain operates on a reward system in which the **ventral tegmental area** (VTA) and **nucleus accumbens,** termed "pleasure centers," release dopamine into the frontal cortex. This chemical elicits a pleasurable sensation and drives motivation and attention. When enormously high levels of dopamine are released by addictive substances or behaviors, the frontal cortex is overwhelmed. Cocaine, for example, increases a person's dopamine levels by 800 percent! After experiencing outrageously high dopamine levels, the brain resets itself and insists upon repeat performances of the substance or behavior; the normal dopamine levels are now interpreted by the brain as being abnormally low, so the brain becomes obsessed with getting more dopamine. Addiction is the ultimate example of taking a good thing too far. Although extraordinarily high dopamine levels play a key role in unhealthy

PLEASURE CENTERS

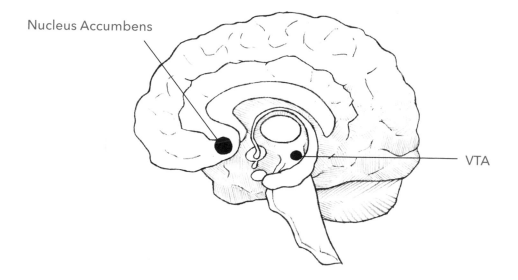

Nucleus Accumbens

VTA

addictive behavior, normal levels of dopamine are not only safe, but they can actually help you in your pursuit of optimal health.

Dopamine is released when you do things you simply enjoy, such as painting a picture, reading a good book, or dancing. Praise increases dopamine levels. Rewards can stimulate the release of dopamine. Even the anticipation of a reward can elevate your dopamine level, which is fortunate because this promotes delayed gratification. The key essentials for the survival and propagation of the human species involve dopamine: exercise, eating, and sex all stimulate the release of dopamine. You'll learn more about this process in Week 9 of The Program. The important thing to understand is that there is chemistry behind motivation that you can tap into in a healthy way as you work on behavior change.

CONCLUSION: *Your brain is motivated by dopamine. Learn to structure your healthy lifestyle around simple things that bring you pleasure. That way, you can promote your motivation to maintain a healthy, sustainable lifestyle.*

7. YOUR SELECTIVE BRAIN

Your brain pays attention to only a small portion of the information it's receiving at any one time. It does this through the **reticular activating system** (RAS), a network of nerve cells that controls consciousness and selective attention to information. The RAS is inactive, for example, when a person is sleeping or under general anesthesia. The frontal cortex still activates in response to incoming information, but the brain neither processes the information nor remembers it. If the RAS is turned on, it will be conscious of the incoming information.

There is a very clever video that was created by Daniel Simons of the University of Illinois and Christopher Chabris of Harvard University several years ago that demonstrates selective attention. It is fun to watch, and I encourage you to take a look at it on the Internet at http://viscog.beckman.uiuc.edu/flashmovie/15.php. In

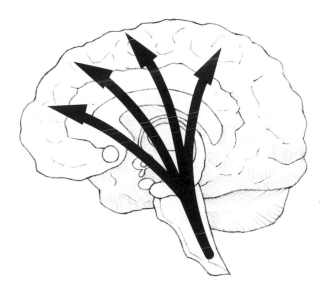

Reticular Activating System

fact, I encourage you to take a look at it now, before you read any further, if you really want a demonstration of what I'm about to describe.

This short video shows how one can fail to see something obvious if concentrating on something else. Technically, your brain does see everything, but it can fail to register all that it sees. In this video clip, the viewer is instructed to count the number of passes a group of adults make to one another with a basketball. There are two balls going at the same time. One point is scored every time a person passes the ball to another person wearing the same color shirt, black or white. More than 50 percent of people who view this video are so preoccupied with counting the passes that they fail to see a gorilla walk right into the center of the group and thump its chest. Now, I've told you the punch line to make my point about selective attention, so if you go online and view this video, you will almost certainly see the gorilla, but ask a colleague or friend to watch the clip. Make sure you emphasize that the point of the exercise is to see if he or she can focus well enough to come up with the accurate number of passes that occur in the video. You will be amazed at how many people miss the gorilla.

A selective brain is efficient. It saves energy. If your brain processed every-thing it saw, heard, smelled, tasted, or felt, it would quickly be overwhelmed with inconsequential information. Selective attention allows you to multitask, to lose yourself in thought without having to expend mental energy on the mundane tasks you do every day. How often have you taken a shower and brushed your teeth in the morning without really thinking about it? How often have you driven to work while lost in thought?

Making a major behavior change often requires that your brain pay atten-tion to behaviors it has become used to ignoring. Change often starts by simply paying close attention to whatever it is you want to change. It may help you to write down what you eat every day, record how many cigarettes you smoke, or list the times you feel anxious. Simply having a heightened consciousness can be pivotal in making a change in your behavior. At first it can be frustrating because what you are doing differently is so new that you keep forgetting to do it. But with practice, as I've said, you will start to remember. Try to build a reminder into your daily routine. After a while, you will not need to make such a conscious effort; your actions will become second nature.

CONCLUSION: *Creating an increased awareness about a particular behavior can make all the difference when it comes to changing that behavior.*

8. YOUR SOCIAL BRAIN

Although we learn from gathering information and from personal experience, we also learn from other people's experiences. Simply hearing a story about some-thing that has happened to another person can set off brain activity that actually mirrors what we would feel if we were having that experience ourselves. The neu-rons that fire in this process are called **mirror neurons,** and they are responsible for our feelings of empathy.

Mirror neurons were first discovered by a group of researchers at the University of Parma in Italy in 1996. This discovery is considered one of the biggest neuroscientific breakthroughs in recent times. It completely changes our understanding of how the brain works. The discovery came through a serendipitous event known as "the raisin incident." Italian scientists were observing a monkey's brain activity during various physical movements. The team decided to take a break. One of the researchers standing near the monkey picked up a raisin and popped it into his mouth. As the monkey watched him, the monkey's brain fired in exactly the same way as if the monkey himself had picked up and eaten the raisin. Simply watching the movement triggered the same brain activity as the actual event. This had never been demonstrated before. In 2005 this same Italian team found that when people listened to stories about other people doing something, the listeners' brains fired as if they themselves were actually doing what was described in the stories.

The scientists went on to discover that mirror neurons do not exist just in premotor areas involved in movement but also in areas of the brain that allow an understanding of someone else's feelings and intentions. In one study, if a person watched a movie in which an actor picked up a teacup and the viewer expected him to drink from the cup, different mirror neurons fired than if the viewer expected the actor to clear the teacup from the table. Different mirror neurons also fire in people when they are shown pictures of faces with varying emotional expressions, such as sadness, happiness, or disgust.

Mirror neurons exist in other animals besides primates. In a 2006 study at McGill University, mice demonstrated empathy for other mice when they saw them in pain. In fact, they themselves experienced pain from a minor stimulus more readily after seeing their cage mates in pain. Interestingly, this finding did not occur if the mice were strangers, only if they knew one another. Actually, if a male (but not a female) mouse encountered a strange male mouse that was experiencing pain, its own pain sensitivity would drop. This would, of course, enhance his ability to win if they started fighting.

Another study, published in *Nature* in 2006, showed that in both men and women, seeing the pain of a person with whom one had just cooperated caused activation of one's own pain pathways. Interestingly, it also showed that if a man (but not a woman) felt that he had been treated unfairly by another man in a previous interaction, his pleasure centers would activate when he saw the other man in pain.

Faulty mirror neurons now appear to explain why those with autism have such a difficult time with language, learning, and empathy. A recent study at Harvard Medical School demonstrated a lack of mirror neurons firing in adolescents suffering from autism. The autistic adolescents could correctly identify the emotions in the facial expressions of the people in the pictures they were shown, but they were not able to empathize with the people in the pictures.

Our ability to learn from one another can give us a powerful edge in the behavior change process. Mirror neurons help us share other people's experiences and are believed to have played a pivotal role in "the great leap forward" humans accomplished fifty thousand years ago, with the development of tools, language, and social skills that enabled the formation of large, complex societies.

Your brain reacts to social interactions. Healthy social relationships have a positive effect on both your mental and physical health. **Oxytocin** is a feel-good chemical that is released during social interaction, promoting social bonding. Oxytocin is released in very high amounts in mothers after they give birth, promoting the development of tight bonding between mom and baby. In men, the chemical equivalent is vasopressin. Pleasant social interactions can also stimulate the release of dopamine and serotonin, other powerful feel-good chemicals.

Human beings are, in fact, intrinsically quite collaborative. We can see an illustration of this in an interesting game called "The Prisoners' Dilemma" in which two players are taken as "prisoners" and placed in separate rooms. The players' brains are monitored for activity as they make decisions. In this game, a player needs to decide at every turn whether he wants to tattle on the other prisoner, essentially earning points at the other player's expense, or to cooperate with the other player, thereby earning fewer points. If the player himself is tattled on by the other prisoner, he will lose points. One of the most interesting discoveries in this study is that the pleasure centers of the brain are activated most when prisoners are collaborating, rather than when they are working against each other, even though working against the other means that they would be earning more points! This is a fascinating and heartening discovery.

CONCLUSION: *The process of behavior change does not need to be a lone venture. We are all on the journey, working to stay healthy in a world that has become more and more challenging. Take advantage of your social brain. You can learn a lot from other people, and they can learn a lot from you.*

9. YOUR RESPONSIVE BRAIN

Environment is a crucial piece of the puzzle when you look at behavior because your brain reacts profoundly to its surrounding environment. One of the main reasons you are not simply predestined for a particular behavior by your genes is that *your environment can turn those genes on or off;* when you learn how to optimize your environment, you learn how to make behavioral change easier and more successful. Certainly, we are all a little different in terms of how our genes respond to various environments, but what is clear is that environment matters.

How big a role do genes have in learning? Is your ability to learn determined purely by your genes? Although genetic predisposition certainly counts, genes do not inevitably predetermine learning capacity.

In a study at Princeton University in 1992, research scientists looked at two different groups of mice. One group was genetically modifying to be intellectually superior by modifying the gene for the glutamate receptor. Glutamate is a brain chemical, a neurotransmitter that is necessary in learning. The smart mice were called Doogie mice (named after the hit TV series of a boy-genius doctor named Doogie). Another group was genetically manipulated to be intellectually impaired, also done by modifying the gene for the glutamate receptor. The smart mice were then raised in standard cages, but the impaired mice were raised in large cages with toys and exercise wheels and with lots of social interaction. At the end of the study, although the intellectually impaired mice were genetically handicapped, they were able to perform just as well as their genetic superiors. This was a real triumph for nurture over nature. Environment does count.

In 1997 a similar study was done by Fred Gage and his colleagues at the Salk Institute, but in this study there was no genetic manipulation. Average mice in one group were raised in standard mouse cages, while average mice in another group were raised in enriched environments. Not only did mice raised in the enriched environments perform better, but their brains were found, on autopsy, to have developed far more nerve connections. In addition, those mice that enjoyed a more favorable environment also produced *new* neurons. This production of new neurons and increased performance happened even in very old mice! Clearly, the impact of the environment can be enormous.

The changing landscape around us today is one of the major forces behind the obesity epidemic. Think about the environment in which we humans evolved over the past millions of years. The world we live in now is a very different place. In modern times, food is everywhere; it is often processed and stripped of nutrients; and now, with all the technology in our day-to-day living, we barely need to move our bodies to survive. If you don't set up your world to cue your brain toward healthful behavior, you'll be working at a distinct disadvantage. Clear the junk food out of your house, remove all ashtrays from sight, place your workout clothes right where you will see them in the morning—it all makes a difference. Don't underestimate the power of your immediate environment on your behavior. Set up the world around you, as much as you can, to trigger your brain toward healthy behavior.

CONCLUSION: *Your environment has a powerful impact on your behavior. Genes are turned on or off based, to a large degree, on what's right around you. Set up your world so that it encourages healthy living.*

10. YOUR BELIEVING BRAIN

"I can do it." This statement sounds so simple, yet it can be quite powerful if you really believe it. Your brain is greatly influenced by whether you believe you can do something. In fact, your confidence in your ability to perform a task is often as important as the actual skill for doing it. Certainly you need the skill, but you also need to believe that you can make it happen.

This concept is called *self-efficacy*. Self-efficacy is different from self-esteem, which refers to your feeling of self-worth. Self-efficacy refers to your belief in your ability to do something. Albert Bandura of Stanford University first introduced this theory of self-efficacy in 1977 in a seminal article entitled "Self-efficacy: Toward a Unifying Theory of Behavioral Change." Since then, countless studies have confirmed the importance of self-efficacy. In 2005 an article in *Health Promotion Practice* reviewed hundreds of studies on just one aspect of self-efficacy: dealing with one's own chronic disease.

In 1979 the researchers Robert S. Weinberg, Daniel Gould, and Allen Jackson tested the concept of self-efficacy on a group of athletes. They picked one group and arbitrarily told each member that he had triumphed in a competition of muscular strength against his competitors. They told each athlete in the other group that he had been outperformed by his competitors. Both groups were then placed in a competition that focused on a motor task measuring physical stamina rather than actual strength. What they found was that the group who had been told their muscle strength was superior displayed significantly more physical stamina than the group who had been told they had previously been outperformed. A higher sense of self-efficacy led to a greater effort, which translated into more success.

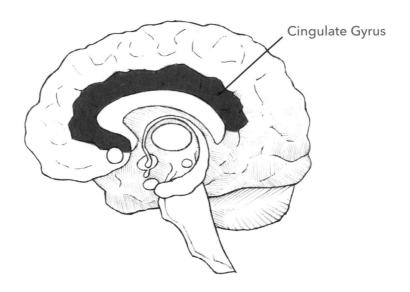

Cingulate Gyrus

In 1988 the researcher Mark D. Litt performed a study on self-efficacy with regard to pain tolerance. A group of people were subjected to painful (cold) stimuli while their ability to endure this pain was monitored. They were then told, arbitrarily, that they had either a high or a low tolerance to pain, regardless of what their performance had been. The subjects were then retested. Those who had been told they had a higher pain tolerance did much better tolerating pain on subsequent tests than those who had been told they had a lower pain threshold. In the next phase of the study, those with a purportedly high pain threshold were given the opposite feedback; they were told that their pain tolerance had dropped. This group then collectively did worse on subsequent pain testing. Although this group's performance dropped after being given negative feedback, its members still retained a higher overall level of self-efficacy and performed better than they had on their initial testing.

In 1990, Thérèse Bouffard-Bouchard and her colleagues tested self-efficacy relative to academic performance. The researchers arbitrarily gave each member of a group of students an evaluation of his or her ability irrespective of their actual performance. Students who were told they had a high ability reported higher self-efficacy, developed more ambitious goals for themselves, demonstrated better problem-solving strategies, and performed better on academic testing than those who were cognitively equal but who had been led to believe they weren't so capable.

It is important to believe in your ability whether you are working on behavior change or anything else, for that matter. If you believe in yourself, you are more likely to set higher goals and are more likely to demonstrate resilience in the face of setbacks. You are consequently more likely to succeed.

How can you believe in yourself, you might ask, when you are filled with negative messages and self-doubts? Often the vision we have of ourselves comes from messages we received during childhood. These messages may have been positive or negative. Perhaps you experienced things that reinforced a negative feeling about yourself. Unfortunately, such a negative concept feeds on itself. If you were told you were clumsy, you are more likely to be clumsy. When you do something that you feel is clumsy, you will likely tell yourself that you really *are* clumsy, and the idea reinforces itself once again. What if you were to switch the message? What if you started telling yourself that you are well coordinated? What if you started telling yourself that you are funny, intelligent, loving, attractive, and healthy? Once you start sending yourself these messages, over time you start to believe them. It becomes a self-fulfilling prophecy. *You tend to be whoever you think you are.* It is important that you understand how powerful this is.

You *can* learn to believe in yourself. Yes, your wonderfully adaptable brain can redefine itself. One of the most powerful ways of doing this is by taking small steps that build, one on top of the other. Each week, you can work on little goals that move you toward your larger goals. The goals should be achievable so that you can actually accomplish them and thereby reinforce your self-efficacy. You can add more small goals the following week. Small successes lead to a higher self-efficacy. This doesn't happen overnight. It requires resending the message over and over, for an extended period of time, but it certainly can be done. Your belief in yourself can and will evolve over your lifetime. The Program is designed around this basic principle.

One of the areas involved in believing is the **cingulate gyrus,** the primitive cortical layer that makes up the outer area of your limbic system. The cingulate gyrus acts as a filter through which information is weighed against that which the brain has previously known to be true. It alerts you when it senses there is something "not quite right" about the information it is receiving. For example, it fires when you hear something that does not jibe with previous information. It also fires when you feel pain or eat something with an unpleasant taste.

Linked to self-efficacy is *goal visualization.* You need to have a clear vision of yourself having achieved the goals you are working toward. Don't underestimate the power of your mind in this. If you want to make a change, you need to have a vision of yourself after you've made the change. If you want to lose 20 pounds, visualize the new, thinner you. If you want to be more at peace with your life, visualize yourself as happy and content.

How do you look in this vision? How do you feel? What are you doing? Remember that goal visualization is more powerful if it is done in the present tense. You influence your brain more if you say, "I am a former smoker. I love breathing clean air into my lungs" than if you say, "I want to stop smoking."

After three decades of research, the concept of self-efficacy continues to be regarded as one of the major forces in behavior change. Believe in yourself. It really does make a difference.

CONCLUSION: *Simply believing in your ability to perform a task is often as important as having the actual skill for doing it.*

11. YOUR EXERCISING BRAIN

Physical exercise changes both the function and physical structure of the brain. The effects of exercise on the brain are truly remarkable. When you move your body in exercise, your muscles churn out several different kinds of growth factors, known as insulin-like growth factor (IGF-1), vascular endothelial growth factor (VEGF-1), and fibroblast growth factor (FGF-2), that drive the brain's production of new building materials that become the infrastructure for new nerve circuits. Exercise also drives the production of brain derived neurotrophic factor (BDNF), which promotes the birth of new, baby neurons, a process called *neurogenesis.* BDNF also supports the growth of already established neurons and nerve networks. Exercise also generates the production of all sorts of feel-good chemicals such as serotonin, norepinephrine, dopamine, endocannabinoids, and endorphins. Your rapidly beating heart also produces atrial natriuretic peptide (ANP), which races over to the brain and directly shuts off the stress response originating in your limbic system. Exercise increases the chemical gamma-aminobutyric acid (GABA), which acts on Valium-like receptors of the brain to promote a more relaxed feeling. The bottom line is this: If you want to learn better, have more energy, be more alert, and feel happier and less stressed, a solid exercise program is always your best bet.

CONCLUSION: *Exercise physically changes your brain. It helps you learn and remember better. It promotes alertness and enhances creative thinking. It elevates mood and lowers stress. In short, exercise is your biggest ally in achieving and maintaining good health.*

12. YOUR UNIQUE BRAIN

One of the greatest things about people is that no two of us are exactly the same. We begin our lives with unique DNA blueprints; we then march through life encountering innumerable experiences that ultimately shape who we become. We all have unique gifts and talents, and we all have unique vulnerabilities and challenges. Each of us views the world in a slightly different way. This is why, in adopting any new lifestyle behavior, you need to go forward in a way that makes sense to you personally. Certainly, it can be helpful to hear about strategies that have worked for other people, but these strategies really matter only if they work for you. There is no "one size fits all" in life or in health. There are many different ways to live a healthy life, and all of the strategies in The Program can be modified to suit each individual person. One thing is for sure: your circumstances will change over time. At one stage of your life, you may find it difficult to get exercise in because you have young children; later, your career may involve travel where you find yourself living out of a suitcase in unfamiliar cities, making exercise even more difficult. Certainly your challenges will change over time, so what you really need to learn is how to stay flexible and solve your problems no matter what situation you find yourself in. How you do this might surprise you. Your solution may not appeal to anyone else, it may not work for anyone else, but as long as it works for you, that's all that matters.

CONCLUSION: *The basic principles of staying healthy may be the same for everyone, but the way you work these principles into your life can be tailored just for you. We all want to be healthy, but how you choose to make this happen has to work for you in your own unique way.*

PART II | THE 12-WEEK PROGRAM

GETTING STARTED

Tell me and I forget, show me and I remember, involve me and I understand.

—ANONYMOUS

WELCOME TO THE PROGRAM! The purpose of this program is to empower you with all of the information and tools you need to live a healthy, happy life. As I said in the introduction, 50 percent of the health problems seen in the United States are due to an unhealthy lifestyle, so learning these tools is important.

You don't need to go to medical school to understand how the human body works, nor do you need a Ph.D. in neuroscience to take advantage of all of the information available today about the brain. You do, however, need to know how to put this information to use, and that is what this book is all about. While The Program delivers all of the latest research, it is designed to deliver the information in a practical way so that you can easily apply it to your everyday life. The Program has worked for thousands of people over the last few years, and with a little effort and commitment on your part, I know it can work for you too.

There are a couple of reasons I'm so confident that The Program will help you. First, all of the information I'm going to give you is based on recent, cutting-edge studies, not only in neuroscience but in the fields of medicine, nutrition, and fitness as well. Although this book is packed with information, if you just remember the major points over the next twelve weeks, you'll have learned everything you need to know. Second, because I've incorporated new knowledge about the brain from the latest research in neuroscience, The Program really works. Why? Because, as I've mentioned, when it comes to making permanent, positive lifestyle changes, your brain can be uncooperative at first. It will resist you, at least in the beginning. It feels comfortable and safe as long as you keep doing everything the way you always have. Tell your brain you want to make a change—say, give up smoking—and it gets nervous, starts to stress, and says, "Not so fast, pal." There are, however, effective ways of coaxing your brain into becoming a better partner, and I've built these methods, or brain tips, right into The Program. Whether your health goal is to lose weight or get fit, reduce stress or boost your mood and energy level, you can use this method to achieve it.

It's not always going to be easy. In fact, I think it can be quite challenging to stay healthy in today's world. It's hard to fit exercise into a life already packed with work, family, and so many other obligations. It's challenging to stay at your ideal weight when there is so much tempting, often unhealthy food everywhere you turn. It's also hard to get enough sleep and manage stress in this fast-paced world. There is so much conflicting information around today, it can even be hard to know what to believe when it comes to healthful living.

As if this weren't enough, our genes and instincts that helped us back when we were tramping around on the savanna sometimes work against us now. Our behavioral instincts have evolved over millions of years and under many conditions that are no longer present today. The world has changed dramatically in a very short period of time, but our brains have not. Did you know that it is estimated that early people had to walk from five to twenty miles every day just to find food? Yet most of us feel annoyed if we have to park more than a few blocks away from our destination. Your body *needs* to move to stay healthy, but your brain has evolved to make you want to conserve energy whenever you can. This made sense millions of years ago, so that you wouldn't foolishly burn calories if you didn't have to; back then, you didn't know when you'd find your next meal. So your brain has evolved to say, "Why walk more than I have to?" Think about this the next time you find yourself desperately searching for the parking spot closest to the grocery store entrance. You are listening to old, outdated brain instincts.

Your brain also wants you to eat food whenever it sees it. That, too, made sense long ago when food was scarce, but most of us aren't in danger of starving anymore. In fact, this instinct has become a big problem in places where the food supply exceeds the actual needs of the population. In the United States, for example, we produce twice as much food each year as we actually need. It is clear that living in a healthful way won't always come naturally since we are wired for a different evolutionary period, but it really *is* necessary if we want to have a long and healthy life.

One of my major goals in The Program is to show you how all the areas of your health are interconnected. That is, you won't be really successful in addressing one health goal without understanding how all the pieces fit together in the big picture of your overall health. Once you understand what is happening with your body and why it matters, you'll be much more successful in meeting your health goals. Also, feel free to talk about The Program with your doctor, especially if you learn about a health issue that you feel pertains particularly to you.

Just as important as learning this information is figuring out how to put it into action in a way that is sustainable. I want you to be able to be healthy for the rest of your life, not just for the twelve weeks you are on The Program. To do this, you need to learn how to adapt the basic principles of health to your own unique lifestyle. You will be given suggestions about what to work on each week, but remember that how you end up working these principles into your life is up to you. Be creative. Make them fit. They have to work only for you. I'm also going to show you how to tailor The Program to your personal goals by teaching you how to be your own best coach. Understanding how to coach yourself is essential if you want to sustain your new, healthful lifestyle. You'll learn exactly how to do this.

Here's how The Program is structured. Each week you'll be given three topics:

health, nutrition, and fitness. At the end of every week, I will list the key points from that week's material, and I'll feature one brain tip. I will also give you a few specific action tasks that pertain to that week's material. It will look like this:

- **Learn It!** This will be a brief summary of the key points in health, nutrition, and fitness from that week.

- **Personalize It!** You will be given one brain tip to focus on, plus a few examples of how past participants in The Program have personalized this brain tip and put it to work in their lives.

- **Live It!** This section will be your "to do" list for the week—a few practical, concrete steps you can take to move forward toward a more healthful life. Feel free to modify these tasks so that they work for you.

You can read this book all in one sitting, or you can read one chapter a week and allow the method to unfold as you go. Either way, you should wait to do the Live It! exercises until they are introduced each week; otherwise, you will be trying to do too much too soon. You can do The Program with a friend or family member or even with a group of friends; doing it together can provide invaluable support and accountability. I encourage you to go online to www.theprogrambook.com to take advantage of the many online features available to you. Here, you can participate in The Program with friends and family, track your exercise, keep a food log, and create weekly goals.

Now let's get started! First, it is important to have a clear picture of your current health, so please answer the Health Risk Assessment Questionnaire that follows. Although your doctor can give you the best assessment of your overall health, you can get a good idea of where you stand from this simple assessment. The scoring is self-explanatory, but no matter how you score, most of us have some room for improvement. Weight, activity, blood pressure, cholesterol, blood sugar, sleep, stress, mood, tobacco, alcohol—all of these count when you look at health. At the end of The Program, take this assessment again to see how much you've improved.

HEALTH RISK ASSESSMENT QUESTIONNAIRE

A LIST QUESTIONS

Do you smoke or use other forms of tobacco?   YES ☐ NO ☐

Do you drink more than one to two glasses
of alcohol per day on average?   YES ☐ NO ☐

B LIST QUESTIONS

Is your blood sugar level above normal?   YES ☐ NO ☐

Is your cholesterol level above normal?   YES ☐ NO ☐

Is your blood pressure above normal?   YES ☐ NO ☐

Do you need to lose more than ten pounds
to be at your ideal weight?   YES ☐ NO ☐

Do you feel your stress level is too high?   YES ☐ NO ☐

Do you feel you suffer from depression or anxiety?   YES ☐ NO ☐

Do you skip your daily thirty minutes of exercise
more than you get it in?   YES ☐ NO ☐

C LIST QUESTIONS

Do you eat junk food (cookies, chips, candy,
soft drinks) most days?   YES ☐ NO ☐

Do you feel fatigued much of the time?   YES ☐ NO ☐

Do you feel your diet is lacking in fruits,
vegetables, and high-fiber grains?   YES ☐ NO ☐

Do you have trouble getting seven to nine hours
of good-quality sleep every night?   YES ☐ NO ☐

Scoring

A List: For every yes, assign 3 points.

B List: For every yes, assign 2 points.

C List: For every yes, assign 1 point.

Add up the points to get your total score.   Total score _____

Interpretation

0–2 points: Generally, your health habits are excellent.

3–5 points: You have good health habits, but they could be improved.

6–9 points: Your health habits need improvement.

10–13 points: Your health habits fall into a high-risk profile.

14–24 points: Your health habits fall into a very-high-risk profile.

In addition to taking the Health Risk Assessment, I encourage you to enter the results of your most recent blood tests or physical examination in Health Stats on page 370 in the Appendix so that you can compare your "before" and "after" results upon completing The Program.

Now it's time to create your health goals. Choose up to three long-term health goals you would like to accomplish. They may be related to weight loss, stress management, higher energy, greater fitness, better sleep habits, healthier eating habits, improved blood pressure, cholesterol or blood sugar, or any other health issue that concerns you. Keep it manageable. Pick no more than three. Make sure your goals are realistic for the twelve-week time period. Don't aim for the impossible. You can always take things to the next level once you reach your initial goal.

Remember, you don't have to do it all at once. In fact, you are more likely to succeed if you approach your goals slowly and gradually.

Long-term Goals

Examples:

- I want to improve my fitness.

- I want to achieve better balance in my life.

- I want to lose ten pounds.

Now create up to three short-term goals you can work on this first week that will advance you in the direction of your long-term goals. Design these goals around the SMART goal format. The goals you define should be:

S = specific
M = measurable
A = action-oriented (behavior-based)
R = realistic
T = time-specific

Short-term Goals for Week 1

Examples:

- I will walk at least half an hour three times this week.

- I will not schedule any work-related meetings or phone calls this week in the evenings so I can spend more time with my family.

- I will not eat any desserts this week.

List three challenges that you predict you will encounter as you work toward your goals, and for each challenge, list a strategy you would be willing to try.

CHALLENGE: I feel too tired to exercise when I get home after work.

STRATEGY: I'll walk Bobby to school instead of driving him. It's good exercise for him, and I can walk the dog at the same time.

CHALLENGE: I know my client will want to meet in the evening for dinner.

STRATEGY: I'll say no but suggest three other times we could meet.

CHALLENGE: It's going to be hard to pass up the doughnuts at work.

STRATEGY: I'll make sure they are set on the table by the back hall so they won't be right in front of me.

People often worry that they will fail because they don't have enough will-power to keep going, but the fact is that achieving your health goals has more to do with having a *good game plan* than with willpower. Your success depends upon devising strategies to address your particular challenges, strategies that will work for you. You may find it helpful to use the goals log in the appendix on page 366.

NUTRITION: LET'S BEGIN WITH THE BASICS

We all know that eating right is one of the most important ways to stay healthy, but we also know that this is not always such an easy thing to do. Information about nutrition always seems to be changing. Just when you think you are making a healthy choice, newspaper headlines call it into question. One day tuna is sitting on top of the health throne, the next day it is said to be loaded with mercury. One day vitamin E is touted as the wellspring of health, preventing heart disease and dementia; then studies come along that fail to bear this out.

The subject of nutrition can certainly seem overwhelming, but it is actually pretty straightforward. I'm going to teach you the fundamentals of healthful nutrition over the next twelve weeks. Eating a healthful diet is one of the most important things you can do for yourself whether you want to lose weight or just stay healthy. Let's start with the basics in order to establish a good foundation.

First, all food is made up of three macronutrients that provide the calories in your diet: **carbohydrates, protein,** and **fat.** In the typical American diet, 50 percent of the daily calories come from carbohydrates, 15 percent from protein, and 35 percent from fat. Fad diets that come and go often argue about the supposed perfect ratio of these macronutrients. Some say protein should represent a higher percentage. Some say carbohydrates should represent a higher percentage. The truth is that there is no perfect ratio. Different cultures all over the world eat differently, and ratios differ considerably. It's not the ratio that indicates whether the diet is healthful. What matters is whether you consume excess calories and whether the macronutrients themselves are of the "good" or "bad" variety. Not all carbohydrates, protein, and fat are created equal. Here's why.

Let's take carbohydrates. Every gram of carbohydrate delivers four calories. Carbohydrates are found in grains such as breads and cereals, as well as in fruits, vegetables, and dairy products. Carbohydrates are also found in treats such as candy and baked goods. The "good" carbohydrates, which are the carbohydrates we should all be predominantly eating, are in the whole-grain form. They are not processed or refined. When you eat a refined, processed product, it has been stripped of nutrients and fiber. Stick with whole-grain breads and cereals. Fruits and vegetables are best when they are in their original form. For example, juicing often removes the valuable fiber of a fruit or vegetable, and cooking can inactivate nutrients as well.

Protein comes from both plant and animal sources. Every gram of protein delivers four calories, the same as a carbohydrate; however, meats and meat substitutes are generally higher in calories per serving than carbohydrate-based foods because protein products usually contain more fat. Animal proteins contain largely saturated fat ("bad fat"), while plant and fish proteins contain largely unsaturated fat ("good fat"). Your best choices for protein are therefore plant products and fish. Poultry and eggs are your next best choice.

While protein and carbohydrates deliver four calories for every gram, fat supplies nine calories for every gram. Because of this, it is easy to get more calories than your body needs if you consume a diet high in fat. Fat is classified as "bad" or "good" based on whether it is saturated or not. Trans fat (an artificially created saturated fat) is particularly bad. Saturated fat and trans fat are considered unhealthy partly because they increase "bad" cholesterol and therefore contribute to heart disease, but also because they contribute to other health risks. (Recent research suggests that saturated fat may not be as big a villain as we once thought, but the recommendation is still to minimize it.)

Many processed junk foods and fast foods contain trans fat, although food manufacturers have started removing trans fat from food products lately because the public has become more aware of its health risks. Fat, however, is not all bad. Fat slows the time it takes for food to leave your stomach after you have eaten, so it keeps you feeling full longer. Unsaturated fats are healthy, partly because they improve your "good" cholesterol level, but also because they provide additional health benefits that we'll go over later.

> 1 gram of carbohydrate = 4 calories
> 1 gram of protein = 4 calories
> 1 gram of fat = 9 calories

There are many other nutrients in food besides carbohydrates, protein, and fat. All have vital roles even though they do not provide calories. These nutrients include water, vitamins, minerals, and phytochemicals. I'll discuss these nutrients in the coming weeks.

The food you eat can be broken into six main food groups. Each group contains different ratios of carbohydrates, protein, and fat. The six food groups are grains, fruits, vegetables, meats and meat substitutes, dairy products, and fats/oils.

- **Grains** are mostly *carbohydrates,* but they contain a little *fat* and *protein.*

- **Fruits** are all *carbohydrates* with only a few exceptions (such as olives and avocados).

- **Vegetables** are mostly *carbohydrates* but also contain a little *protein.*

- **Meats** are a mixture of *protein* and *fat.* **Meat substitutes** are generally plant-based, made from nuts, seeds, beans, and lentils. Beans and lentils are generally low in fat, while nuts and seeds are high in fat; although the fat in nuts is healthy, the number of calories in each serving is quite high, so watch portions carefully.

- **Dairy** products are a combination of *carbohydrates, protein,* and *fat.* They are actually quite high in fat, and because the fat is from an animal, it is of the unhealthy, saturated type. Try to get your dairy products in nonfat form when possible.

- **Fats and oils** are 100 percent fat.

- **Sweets and treats** aren't actually a food group, but they can be thought of as the seventh food category. They are made up of sugar or refined carbohydrates. Large amounts of saturated fats and trans fats are often found in these foods as well. Examples include cakes, cookies, chips, and candy.

To put this in a way that may be even easier to understand, take a look at "Meet the Food Groups," which shows you the breakdown of macronutrients in all the basic food groups.

MEET THE FOOD GROUPS

GRAINS

- Bread (15% protein, 70% carbohydrate, 15% fat)

- Cereal (15% protein, 70% carbohydrate, 15% fat)

- Pasta (17% protein, 75% carbohydrate, 8% fat)

- Rice (10% protein, 85% carbohydrate, 5% fat)

FRUITS

- All fruit is 100% carbohydrate, except:

  - Avocado* (12.5% protein, 12.5% carbohydrate, 75% fat)

  - Olive* (15% protein, 85% fat)

VEGETABLES

- All vegetables are approximately 90% carbohydrate, 10% protein

MEAT OR MEAT SUBSTITUTES

- Lean beef (40% protein, 60% fat)

- Pork (45% protein, 55% fat)

- Lamb (55% protein, 45% fat)

- Chicken with skin (60% protein, 40% fat)

- Chicken without skin (75% protein, 25% fat)

- Turkey with skin (60% protein, 40% fat)

- Turkey without skin (80% protein, 20% fat)

- Fish:

  - Salmon (60% protein, 40% fat)

  - Red snapper (85% protein, 15% fat)

- Beans and lentils (25% protein, 75% carbohydrate)

- Chickpeas/garbanzo beans (20% protein, 65% carbohydrate, 15% fat)

- Soybeans (30% protein, 30% carbohydrate, 40% fat)

- Tofu (40% protein, 10% carbohydrate, 50% fat)

- Nuts* and seeds* (15% protein, 15% carbohydrate, 70% fat)

- Peanut butter* (15% protein, 15% carbohydrate, 70% fat)

- Egg (40% protein, 60% fat)

DAIRY

- Whole milk (20% protein, 30% carbohydrate, 50% fat)

- Nonfat milk (40% protein, 60% carbohydrate, 0% fat)

- Whole-milk yogurt (15% protein, 75% carbohydrate, 10% fat)

- Nonfat yogurt (25% protein, 75% carbohydrate, 0% fat)

- Cheese* (25% protein, 75% fat)

- Low-fat cheese (50% protein, 50% fat)

- Sour cream* (7.5% protein, 7.5% carbohydrate, 85% fat)

- Nonfat sour cream (25% protein, 75% carbohydrate)

- Cream cheese* (10% protein, 90% fat)

- Nonfat cream cheese (70% protein, 30% carbohydrate)

- Cream* (100% fat)

- Whole-milk cottage cheese (50% protein, 15% carbohydrate, 35% fat)

- Nonfat cottage cheese (80% protein, 20% carbohydrate, 0% fat)

FATS AND OILS

- Vegetable oils* (100% fat)

- Butter* (100% fat)

SWEETS AND TREATS

- Cookie (5% protein, 55% carbohydrate, 40% fat)

- Cake (5% protein, 50% carbohydrate, 45% fat)

- Chocolate bar (5% protein, 45% carbohydrate, 50% fat)

- Hard candy (100% carbohydrate)

- Brownie (5% protein, 65% carbohydrate, 30% fat)

- Pastry (5% protein, 40% carbohydrate, 55% fat)

- Doughnut (5% protein, 50% carbohydrate, 45% fat)

- Whole-milk ice cream* (5% protein, 25% carbohydrate, 70% fat)

- Nonfat frozen yogurt (15% protein, 85% carbohydrate)

* Any food containing 70% or more fat is often regarded as a "fat." Examples include cheese, nuts, avocados, olives, peanut butter, sour cream, cream, cream cheese, ice cream.

Next week, I'll go over the food groups in more detail to help you design your own personal nutritional plan, but here are two things you can do this week.

1   **Start keeping a food log of everything you eat each day.** This can be an extremely valuable tool. Whether you want to lose weight or simply develop better eating habits, a food log will help raise your consciousness regarding your eating patterns. It will help you identify what, when, where, why, and how you eat. Take the time to do this. It will make a big difference.

   This may seem tedious at first, but many studies show that food and exercise logs are one of the most powerful tools in behavior change. Tracking creates a heightened awareness that stimulates your powerful frontal cortex (the area in your brain devoted to higher, complex thinking) to become more engaged in behaviors that have become automatic and reflexive.

   Some people find that tracking for just the first few weeks is all they really need to jump-start their awareness, but others find it helps to continue tracking over the long haul. You decide. For the first few weeks of The Program, however, I urge everyone to keep a log. An example of a food log is included in the Appendix on page 365, but feel free to use any method of tracking that works for you. You can track other things, too: you can track your weight if you are working on weight loss; you can track your mood if you are working on feeling happier or less stressed.

2   **Remove all the junk food from your house.** The less junk food kept in the house, the easier it is to eat healthfully. If for some reason you feel you cannot remove the junk food from your house—for instance, if a family member insists that it stay— put it all in one cupboard of the kitchen, in an out-of-sight, hard-to-reach location. Stock the house with healthful, easy-to-grab snacks such as cut fresh fruit and veggies, low-fat string cheese, nonfat yogurt, and low-fat, high-fiber energy bars. The easier it is to eat healthful food, the more likely it is to happen.

   In this first week, don't worry about following any specific dietary plan. That will come next week. Just try to eliminate sweets and treats from your diet. If you are really eager to get started on a specific nutrition plan, though, you can read ahead to Week 2.

FITNESS: THE IMPORTANCE OF BEING FIT

One major theme that runs throughout The Program is the importance of physical activity to health. Whatever health goals you may have, the importance of a regular exercise program cannot be overstated. *Our bodies are wired to move.* At a cellular level, things start to go awry when we stop moving our bodies.

There are three components of fitness: *cardiorespiratory, strength,* and *flexibility.* I'll go over each of these in detail throughout the coming weeks, but all three components play a role in keeping one healthy.

A solid exercise program consists of 30 to 60 minutes of moderate- to high-intensity aerobic activity most days of the week, with 5 minutes of flexibility exercises daily and two or three 15-minute sessions per week of resistance exercises, particularly targeting the five big core muscles of your body: your chest, abdomen, back, shoulders, and thighs. This may sound daunting at first, but it really isn't once you get into the swing of it.

Why Be Fit?

Exercise can boost your metabolic rate by as much as 20 to 30 percent.

One question I'm asked all the time is: What is the minimum amount one has to do to stay healthy? Come on, admit it, you were wondering that too. Well, you could get the very minimum amount of exercise you need each day by walking for a half hour. You should walk at a brisk clip for the exercise to be intense enough, and you really need to do it every day. It's okay if you miss a day here or there, but try to do it every day. That is the minimum we all need to do to begin to tap into the health benefits of exercise and see a reduction in disease. More exercise, however, will increase the benefits you reap.

For most resistance exercises, you really don't need any special equipment other than your own body. In The Program, we do present some exercises that use a resistance band. A band is easily obtained online or at any sporting goods store for about $10. No matter what you do, though, *keep it simple.* That's the major message I want you to hear.

Flexibility exercises are easy and require no special equipment. You should do them when your body temperature is warm, so an ideal time is right after you finish your aerobic activity. You could also do flexibility exercises first thing after a warm shower or bath.

Physical activity helps to achieve virtually any health goal you may be working toward, so let me explain exactly why exercise is so important to good health.

First, having a regular exercise program is the most important predictor not only of weight loss but also of weight maintenance. Of people who have lost significant amounts of weight and kept it off over the long haul, more than 90 percent engage in regular exercise, with walking being the most popular mode of exercise and 270 minutes being the average total amount of time spent exercising each week. This translates into about 40 minutes a day or 60 minutes four to six days per week. It is extremely helpful to keep an up-to-date exercise log in plain view so that you can stay realistic at all times about your progress.

Physical activity also significantly reduces your risk of developing heart disease. People without known heart disease who exercise even modestly but on a regular, consistent basis are significantly less likely to suffer from heart disease and more likely to live longer lives. People who have already had a heart attack who walk for 30 minutes a day have an 80 percent increase in survival rate.

Physical activity reduces your risk of developing diabetes. When you exercise, your muscles release growth factors that stimulate an increased production of insulin receptors; these growth factors also help your circulating insulin work more efficiently. By improving the sensitivity of your cells' insulin receptors, you can either avoid developing diabetes or, if you already have diabetes, achieve better control of it.

Exercise also stimulates the immune system, so people who exercise on a regular basis are less likely to get infections.

The risk of developing certain cancers, in particular breast and colon cancers, is reduced in those who exercise regularly. Regular exercise has been shown to decrease the risk of breast cancer by 50 percent and colon cancer by 60 percent.

Memory is improved by aerobic exercise through an increase in BDNF, brain-derived neurotrophic (nerve growth) factor. You actually make more brain cells when you exercise! Imagine that! In the elderly, regular exercise lowers the incidence of dementia. At a chemical level, when you exercise, your muscles release growth factors, which migrate to the brain and activate genes that produce proteins necessary for building the new infrastructure for *new* nerve networks. This is one of the most remarkable new discoveries about the brain.

Exercise increases mental alertness. When you exercise, you produce more neurotransmitters such as norepinephrine and dopamine. These chemicals increase your attention and motivation. The effect seems to be highest in the first couple of hours after you exercise, but if you exercise on a regular basis, you will find that you are more alert in general.

Mood is enhanced by regular exercise. When you exercise, the brain's release of serotonin facilitates a calmer, happier mood.

Regular exercise often decreases chronic pain from any source. This is because exercise increases the release of endorphins, endocannabinoids, and serotonin, all of which increase a person's pain threshold. Exercise also reduces joint pain from arthritis because it stimulates an increase in the production of synovial fluid, which bathes and lubricates the joints.

Sleep is greatly improved by regular exercise. Exercise accentuates your natural body temperature swings throughout the day, and this increases the amount of time you spend in the deeper, more restorative stages of sleep, stages three and four. It is in these deeper stages of sleep that you release vital chemicals that stimulate your immune system and repair the ongoing wear and tear of daily living.

Exercise is one of the best ways to manage stress. When you exercise, your rapidly beating heart releases a chemical called atrial natriuretic peptide (ANP), which crosses over to the brain and directly turns off the stress response. Exercise also elevates calming endorphins and endocannabinoids and the calming feel-good chemical serotonin, which I've mentioned before. Exercise not only turns the stress response off, it gives you a longer fuse, so the stress response doesn't activate as easily in the first place.

Weight-bearing exercise promotes bone strength and decreases the chance of developing osteoporosis so that fracture risk is reduced. Fractures are also reduced because core muscle strength is improved. This leads to better balance and fewer falls among the elderly.

Finally, it has been shown that people who exercise regularly not only enjoy longer lives but also have higher-quality lives than those who remain sedentary. Now, that's pretty tough to beat!

LEARN IT!

- All areas of your health are interconnected.

- Fifty percent of all health problems can be prevented by a healthy lifestyle.

- Your brain resists sudden change but accepts gradual change.

- All foods are made up of three macronutrients: carbohydrates, protein, and fat.

- 1 gram of carbohydrate = 4 calories; 1 gram of protein = 4 calories; 1 gram of fat = 9 calories.

- "Good" carbohydrates are unprocessed; "bad" carbohydrates have been processed and stripped of fiber and other nutrients.

- "Good" proteins are either low in fat or contain unsaturated fats; "bad" proteins are high in saturated fat.

- "Good" fats are unsaturated; "bad" fats are either naturally or artificially saturated.

- Your body is wired to move. Exercise is *essential* to good health.

- The minimum amount of exercise needed to stay healthy is 30 minutes on average each day.

- Physical fitness improves mood, alertness, energy, and the ability to learn. It decreases health risks by preventing infections, cancers, heart disease, diabetes, obesity, and dementia, to name a few.

PERSONALIZE IT!

This week, work on your Selective Brain.

Your brain does not consciously process all of the information it is exposed to on a daily basis; it is selective. Selective attention allows your brain to think while being on autopilot, therefore letting you do something else; but it can also allow unhealthy behaviors without your even being aware you are doing them. Change often starts by simply paying close attention to whatever behavior you would like to change.

Here are some examples of how people in The Program have personalized this brain principle and put it into action.

- Shelby T., a 45-year-old venture capitalist, wrote down her goals and kept them by the parking brake of her car, so every time she drove anywhere she could remind herself of her goals and behaviors she was working on. These constant reminders helped keep her goals uppermost in her mind.

- Alice Y., a 26-year-old law student, set up her computer to text-message herself several times a day as a reminder to keep a food journal because she frequently grazed all day without thinking about it. Eventually she became conscious of her eating behavior without these constant reminders.

- Nick S., a 51-year-old biology professor, kept a spreadsheet on his computer of how many miles he had accumulated daily on his pedometer so he could see at a glance how he was doing on his exercise goals. The simple act of tracking his miles every day gave his daily exercise a higher priority level and he was more likely to make time for it.

LIVE IT!

- Take the Health Risk Assessment to get a clear picture of where your health currently stands. Fill out the Health Stats form in the Appendix, page 370.

- Create three long-term health goals for The Program and three short-term goals for this week.

- Clear out the junk food from your cupboards and stock up on healthful food.

- Begin tracking your daily food intake and exercise, and think of ways you can set up regular reminders for yourself regarding your goals.

- Start moving. If you have been sedentary for a long time, you may want to start by walking for 10 minutes a day, working your way up to 30 minutes. You can also divide your cardio exercise into three 10-minute sessions each day to meet the 30-minute daily goal.

CREATING YOUR PERSONAL PLAN

The secret to getting ahead is getting started.

—AGATHA CHRISTIE

WELCOME TO WEEK 2! This week I'm going to help you create your own personal nutrition and exercise plan, and I'm also going to introduce you to your own personal coach: *you.* Becoming your own best coach is probably the most helpful thing you can do for yourself both in The Program and in life. Once you have developed and honed this skill, it can help you be the best you can be at *anything*—not only when working on your health but also in your career, your personal relationships, and any other goals you may have.

Here are the key coaching principles for you to keep in mind and work on as you go through The Program. Let's begin with the most fundamental of coaching concepts, the fact that you can change and grow.

You are entirely capable of changing for the better. As I've mentioned before, your brain is intrinsically wired to allow change. Although the brain may resist sudden, major change, gradual changes are an inevitable part of life, and your brain is okay with that. In truth, all experiences influence the brain and you have new experiences every day. You continue to learn and change throughout your life. As I explained in part I, when you change, your brain physically rewires itself. Isn't that amazing? The fact that you can and do change, at any age, is incredibly empowering. You are not predestined to be any certain way at all. You have a lot of control over who you are and who you will become, even after you've taken your genes into account. Your brain is incredibly adaptable, and so are you.

A good coach helps you develop resilience; this is especially important as you work on behavior change. Setbacks and failures are not necessarily bad; they are part of the process. Setbacks can make you stronger. As you learn and grow and begin to change in The Program, of course you will hit bumps in the road. Everybody does. You will inevitably fall from time to time, but falling down and getting right back up are an essential part of the learning process. Through it, you learn how to be resilient. Sure, it's easy to shine when everything is going well, but when things aren't going the way you planned, *resilience* and *perseverance* are the essential traits that will get you back on track. So don't be afraid to fail. In fact, if you never fail, it is almost certainly a reflection of the fact that you are not pushing yourself to try new things. It may sound like a cliché, but you do learn from your mistakes. As you may remember from part I, studies clearly show that your brain processes information differently when it encounters the very same situation in which you previously made a mistake. Almost everyone who ultimately makes a significant change has made previous attempts and had previous failures before succeeding. Just accept this fact and be willing to get back up and start again. Confucius asked, "How does a man walk a thousand miles? He takes one step at a time."

Another important coaching skill is the ability to *reframe* the way you look at a situation so that you can see it in a positive light. I'm not suggesting that you be unrealistic in a bad situation, but in everything that happens to us there is something positive—even in the toughest times.

It isn't always easy to do this. Sometimes terrible things happen, but from this you can learn that you have an inner strength that will allow you to get through it. And sometimes you actually find that you can benefit from a bad situ ation. For example, Richard, a 49-year-old account executive at an ad agency, lost his job during a major layoff at his company. At first he was devastated. Within a day, though, he had begun to spin it around; he started to see the positive side of what had originally seemed pretty gloomy. In truth, he had not been happy in his job for some time, and the layoff forced him to reevaluate what he was really looking for in his career. What he really wanted to do was teach. Within a month he had found a job at a local university teaching business and management classes to undergraduate students. Looking back, he says, getting laid off was the best thing that ever happened to him.

As you coach yourself, understand that *the biggest driving force for change must come from within you,* not from external forces. Just as you can't force other people to change, neither can anyone force you to change. Your family and friends can certainly be influential in helping you, but that's all they can do. The real work has to come from you.

Certainly, a lot of things in life can get in the way of change. There is too much stress, too little time, too much work, too little play. But if we wait until life calms down before we work on change, it will probably never happen. Your life may indeed calm down for a little while, but then something else will inevitably come along to distract you.

There will be times in your life, however, when it may be easier to change than others. You may hear a message at one point in your life and do nothing about it, but then you hear the same message a few years later and you decide to take action. This point in time is called a *teachable moment.* You are ready.

Change does not happen overnight; it comes in stages. You may be familiar with Dr. James Prochaska's Stages of Change. In 1994, after decades of clinical research, the University of Rhode Island's Dr. Prochaska developed a model to reflect the stages people pass through as they work toward change. The stages go like this:

Precontemplation: "I don't need to change."

Contemplation: "I need to make a change, but I'm not interested in doing it now."

Preparation: "I'm thinking about change and learning about how to do it."

Action: "I'm actively working on making changes now."

Maintenance: "I've made the change and am now in a 'keep going' mode."

Where you lie in the Stages of Change predicts your likelihood of change. For example, using this model, Dr. Prochaska found only a 6 percent success rate for giving up smoking over an eighteen-month period for those who were Precontemplators at the start of the period, compared with a 24 percent success rate for those who were in the Preparation phase.

Know where you are in the Stages of Change progression, and start the process wherever you are. If you aren't ready to change yet, that's okay. Learn what The Program has to teach you, and you will be that much more prepared to take action when you are ready.

A good coach helps you find the things you can change and work around the things you cannot. For example, you can optimize your immediate environment so that it has a positive influence on your behavior. As I've mentioned before, the environment stimulates or suppresses the production of genes that produce the proteins that regulate your behavior. Never underestimate the power of your environment.

Last week, you cleaned out your food cupboards and stocked up on healthful food. This week, look around for other things in your home or work environment that you may want to change. Also, be selective about the people you spend your time with. People are an important part of your environment. We are, after all, very social creatures, and our behavior is strongly influenced by the people around us. In fact, the three questions a person asks before adopting a new behavior are:

- What are the benefits and consequences of doing (or not doing) this?

- Am I capable of doing (or not doing) this?

- *What is everyone else around me doing?*

We watch what everyone around us is doing, and we are more inclined to do something when we see that everybody else is doing it. For example, a 2008 study disclosed that although Americans are more overweight than ever before, they are less able to recognize when they are overweight than they used to be. Everything is relative; you compare yourself to what you see around you. Another 2008 study showed that people are much more likely to eat more when those around them are eating large amounts of food, yet those same people do not feel they are being influenced by those around them. Are there people you socialize with who make it difficult for you to stay healthy? If so, maybe it's time to do something about that.

A good coach recognizes that you are unique and that *different strategies work for different people.* The trick here is to find what works for you in your own individual way. The strategies that work for one person are not necessarily the strategies that will work for someone else. It can be very helpful to hear ideas that have worked for other people, but a good coach knows you may have to tweak those ideas to fit them into your life.

A good coach encourages you to practice goal visualization, which is the ability to visualize yourself having already achieved the goals you are working toward. When your brain gets used to seeing this new, improved you, it starts to believe it is the real you. Whatever your brain believes, your brain acts out. Just as a business must have a plan, a vision of where it is going and what it wants to become, so must you have a vision of yourself having already achieved your goals. The more your brain sees you in a certain way, the more your brain believes that this vision is reality. It's like a dress rehearsal that allows your brain to get used to accepting this image as the real you. If you visualize yourself speaking in public and looking great, acting confident and gregarious, when you actually get up to speak in front of an audience your brain will be so used to seeing you this way, it will behave accordingly. Your thoughts and daydreams are a part of your brain's experiences and part of who your brain believes you to be. The more you visualize yourself having achieved your goals, the more your brain decides that this is the real you and the more it works to promote the behavior that drives this to be true. Use this brain feature to your advantage as much as you can.

Learn to make peace with your imperfections. If I had to pick one and only one coaching principle as the most important, this is the one I would choose. I've worked with thousands of patients, and it always amazes me that so many people are so hard on themselves. They are often their own worst critic. As you move through The Program (and through life, for that matter), remember that you are not doing yourself a favor by constantly criticizing yourself whenever you do something you don't like. If you constantly send yourself negative messages about what you've done wrong, you are essentially telling your brain, over and over again, to create a negative image of yourself. What does your brain do when it hears a message over and over? That's right, it acts the message out. So not only are you not helping yourself when you send yourself negative messages, you are actually working against yourself. *Focus on how you are improving,* not on the fact that you've made some mistakes. Enjoy the whole of who you are, complete with strengths and gifts, as well as challenges and vulnerabilities.

Work on making changes one step at a time. As I've mentioned before, small changes are easier to adopt, and small changes can ultimately lead to big out-comes. A good coach emphasizes the value and power of *gradual change.* There is no question about it: small changes made incrementally over a long period of time can have enormous consequences. Sure, it takes a bit of diligence to plod patiently along without a lot of drama or fanfare, but that's the beauty of it. Before long, you have lost 60 pounds! Or you no longer need your blood pressure or cho-lesterol pills. Or you have become more fit, with a lot more energy and a lot less stress. I know everyone prefers instant results, but if you want your brain to be on board with your efforts, approach change slowly and gradually. And make sure you celebrate all those small, triumphant steps along the way.

NUTRITION: CREATING YOUR PERSONAL NUTRITION PLAN

Last week we discussed the basics of nutrition. This week I want to talk to you about how to apply that knowledge to your own personal goals. What are your nutrition goals? The first question to ask yourself is whether you need to lose weight. A healthy weight is one that falls into a body mass index (BMI) range of less than 25. You can figure out your BMI by going to www.nhlbisupport.com/bmi or the BMI chart in the appendix on page 368. You can find out where you stand by looking at the BMI/weight chart below.

BMI charts certainly aren't perfect. They are designed more for large epidemiologic studies than as a perfect assessment of your ideal weight. For example, large-framed, muscular men may have a higher BMI than "normal" without being overweight. On the other hand, you may be in the "normal" BMI range but still need to lose a little weight. That is, you may still have more body fat than is considered healthy, even with a normal BMI. If you aren't sure, you can check your body fat percentage. A woman's body fat should typically be less than 25 percent and a man's less than 20 percent. Here are the standard BMI/weight status categories for adults.

BMI	WEIGHT STATUS
Below 18.5	Underweight
18.5–24.9	Normal
25.0–29.9	Overweight
30.0 and above	Obese

As you can see, according to the Centers for Disease Control and Prevention, an adult who has a BMI between 25 and 29.9 is considered overweight. An adult with a BMI of 30 or higher is considered obese.

After you have chosen a weight goal, subtract this weight from your current weight to get the number of pounds you need to lose to reach this goal. To lose a pound of fat (not water weight), you need to accumulate a 3,500-calorie deficit. Your weight will stay the same if the calories you take in are equal to the calories you burn.

How do you know how many calories you need to maintain your current weight? There are complicated formulas to figure out how many calories you need, but an easy rule of thumb is to multiply your weight by a factor of 11. If you are younger than 30 years old, you can multiply by 12. This is the number of calories you should consume each day to maintain your current weight. If you exercise, you can add the number of calories you burn to the calories you can eat and your weight will stay the same. An average person burns 200 calories for every 30 minutes of a brisk walk. If the same person jogs, he or she burns 300 calories in the same time. See Exercise and Calorie Expenditure (page 68) for a more detailed summary. The formula I have outlined is not exact, but it is pretty close. To lose weight, you simply need to take in fewer calories than your body needs. The rub is that everybody is a little different. Some people's bodies are highly efficient at getting by with very little fuel coming in each day. By efficient, I mean that their metabolism is low and they don't need many calories to survive. That's great if they live where food is scarce (they'll be the ones who survive), but in today's world, this type of efficiency makes it harder to avoid becoming overweight. If you feel this describes you, rest assured that you certainly can have a normal healthy body weight with this type of metabolism, but it will be even more important for you to exercise on a regular basis. That's okay because everyone should be exercising, but for you, exercise will be crucial for weight control.

To lose a pound in a week, you need to average a deficit of 500 calories per day (or 3,500 calories per week). You lose pounds quickly in the beginning of a diet, but the extra loss is usually due to water loss, not fat loss. In order to lose a true pound, you need to either consume 3,500 fewer calories or burn off 3,500 calories with extra exercise. The best weight loss method is to lose weight at a rate of one to two pounds per week. If you lose much faster than this, your metabolism will slow down. Ouch! You don't want that! And if you lose a lot of fat too quickly, your body will stop taking the calorie deficit out of your fat stores and start taking it from your muscle stores instead. You don't want that either. Your muscle stores are what actually drive your metabolism up, so losing muscle will mean you will need even fewer calories in the future to maintain that weight. That is why dieters who lose weight quickly often gain the weight right back *plus* some extra pounds. Aim for a steady one- to two-pound loss each week so you will minimize your muscle loss.

Also, it's important to realize that you will enjoy quite a number of health benefits simply by losing 5 to 10 percent of your body weight. So even if you can't make it below a BMI of 25, you should still try to get as close to this as you can.

The best way to achieve a 3,500- to 7,000-calorie deficit per week is to reduce your daily caloric intake while you increase your activity. Exercise will help you reach your weight goals much faster. In addition, there are so many other benefits of exercise, some that have already been mentioned and some that we will go over in detail later.

Below is a list that shows you various types of activities and the corresponding calories they expend. These values are based on a 150-pound person doing each of the following activities for 30 minutes. If you weigh more than 150 pounds, you will burn more calories than this list shows. If you have more muscle mass, you will burn more calories for any given exercise. Finally, if you are simply more fit, you will burn more calories. For example, if you are a long-distance runner, your body will burn more calories than someone else of the same weight who is not as fit.

Exercise and Calorie Expenditure

The following values reflect calories expended by a *150-pound person* doing the following activities for *30 minutes:*

Golfing, with cart	100 calories
Bowling	120 calories
Yoga	140 calories
Heavy housecleaning	160 calories
Badminton	160 calories
Low-impact aerobics	175 calories
Stationary cycling (low setting)	175 calories
Golfing, carrying bag	175 calories
Gardening, general	175 calories
Inline blading	175 calories
Dancing	175 calories
Horseback riding	175 calories
Walking, briskly (4 mph)	200 calories
Skiing, downhill	200 calories
Road cycling, leisurely (10 mph)	210 calories
Tennis, social	225 calories
Circuit training	235 calories
Swimming, slow	250 calories
Racquetball	250 calories
Cross-country skiing, light	250 calories
Weight training	275 calories
Basketball	275 calories
Walking/jogging (5 mph)	300 calories
Swimming, fast	350 calories
Road cycling, vigorous (15 mph)	350 calories
Running (10-minute mile or 6 mph)	350 calories

Ski machine	350 calories
Rowing machine (medium)	370 calories
Jumping rope (100 skips per minute)	375 calories
Cross-country skiing, heavy	400 calories
Running (8-minute mile or 7.5 mph)	425 calories

Now that you understand how weight loss and calorie deficits work, it's time to select your Personal Nutrition Plan. In your plan, you will be given a certain number of servings from each of the food groups so that you will be sure to get all the nutrients you need. It's true that you will maintain (or lose) weight based on how many calories are coming in and how many are going out, but calorie reduction isn't everything! You want to stay healthy, so although you can lose weight on a cupcake or beer diet if you are taking in fewer calories than your body needs, a diet like that certainly won't keep you healthy.

Personal Nutrition Plan*

- **The 1,200-calorie plan** is designed for women who don't exercise, don't work in physically demanding environments, and are postmenopausal and/or 55 years or older. If you are too hungry on the 1,200-calorie plan, you may want to move up to the 1,400-calorie plan and add some exercise.

- **The 1,400-calorie plan** is most often used by women who lead active lives, exercise on a regular basis, and are younger than 55 years old. This plan works well for most women.

- **The 1,600-calorie plan** is good for women who are over five feet, seven inches tall and exercise regularly. It also works for a sedentary man.

- **The 1,800-calorie plan** is recommended for men who are active and less than six feet tall.

*You lucky people who are over six feet tall get to eat more. Add one more serving each of grains and dairy products to boost your calorie count closer to 2,000.

The table below shows how many servings of each food group are allocated to the different calorie levels. I will explain serving sizes next. Do your best to stay within the suggested guidelines. By keeping a food log, you will be able to keep track of what you are eating during the day. If you overeat at one meal, do your best to get back on track at your next meal.

	1,200 CALORIES	1,400 CALORIES	1,600 CALORIES	1,800 CALORIES
GRAINS	5 servings	6 servings	7 servings	8 servings
VEGETABLES	4 servings	4 servings	4 servings	4 servings
FRUITS	2 servings	3 servings	3 servings	3 servings
DAIRY	2 servings	2 servings	2 servings	2 servings
MEAT OR MEAT SUBSTITUTES	2 servings	2 servings	2 servings	3 servings
FAT	2 servings	3 servings	4 servings	4 servings

A Personal Nutrition Plan also works for those who just want to eat more healthful foods and don't need to lose any weight. In this case, the Personal Nutrition Plan simply needs to match the number of calories needed for weight maintenance. As I've mentioned, you can find out how many calories you need for weight maintenance by using the "weight (in pounds) times 11" rule. For example, a person who weighs 150 pounds would multiply 150 by 11 and get 1,650. That is the number of calories this person should eat per day to maintain his or her weight, assuming that he or she is not exercising (which would burn additional calories). If you don't need to lose weight, ask yourself if you should improve your eating habits anyway. Take the Rate Your Plate Quiz to find out.

RATE YOUR PLATE QUIZ

In general, do you . . .

Eat regular meals (breakfast, lunch, and dinner) rather than skipping?	USUALLY ☐	SOMETIMES ☐	NEVER ☐
Eat until satisfied but avoid overeating?	USUALLY ☐	SOMETIMES ☐	NEVER ☐
Choose nutritious snacks instead of junk food?	USUALLY ☐	SOMETIMES ☐	NEVER ☐
Include a variety of foods in your diet?	USUALLY ☐	SOMETIMES ☐	NEVER ☐
Choose whole grains instead of processed, refined grains?	USUALLY ☐	SOMETIMES ☐	NEVER ☐
Eat at least three servings of vegetables daily?	USUALLY ☐	SOMETIMES ☐	NEVER ☐
Eat at least two servings of fruit daily?	USUALLY ☐	SOMETIMES ☐	NEVER ☐
Choose nonfat or low-fat dairy products?	USUALLY ☐	SOMETIMES ☐	NEVER ☐
Avoid fried food, fast food, and high-fat foods (such as butter, cream, whole milk)?	USUALLY ☐	SOMETIMES ☐	NEVER ☐
Avoid sweets (candy, cookies, cakes, pies)?	USUALLY ☐	SOMETIMES ☐	NEVER ☐
Stay well hydrated by drinking water instead of high-sugar beverages?	USUALLY ☐	SOMETIMES ☐	NEVER ☐
Limit your consumption of alcoholic beverages?	USUALLY ☐	SOMETIMES ☐	NEVER ☐

Add up your score:

Never = 0 point

Sometimes = 1 point

Usually = 2 points

If you scored:

24 or more points: Healthful eating seems to be your habit already. There is always room for improvement. Try to find ways you can do even better!

16 to 23 points: You are on the right path to healthful eating. With a few easy changes, your eating pattern can be more healthful.

9 to 15 points: You are sometimes on track but not often enough. Your health depends on your making some changes in the nutritional arena.

0 to 8 points: You will benefit greatly from some dietary changes. With small steps and the right support, you can become a much healthier you.

Of course, knowing the number of serving sizes in your Personal Nutrition Plan won't help if you don't know how much a serving size is, so let's go over that right now. Serving sizes are based on easy-to-visualize units to help you keep track so you can be sure you are roughly getting enough of each food group. It isn't important that every day be perfectly balanced, but over time a healthy, balanced diet should be the goal.

SERVING SIZES AT A GLANCE

FOOD GROUP	CALORIES	ONE SERVING EQUALS
Grains	80 calories per serving	1 slice whole-wheat bread 1/2 cup cooked rice or pasta 1/2 cup couscous or potatoes 1/2 English muffin 1/2 mini bagel 1/2 large pita bread 1/2–1 cup cereal 1/4 cup beans, lentils, or legumes
Fruits	60 calories per serving	1 piece fruit 1 cup fresh fruit 1/2 cup canned fruit 1/4 cup dried fruit 1/2 cup fruit juice 1/2 cup applesauce 1/2 medium banana
Vegetables	25 calories per serving	1 cup raw vegetables 1/2 cup cooked vegetables
Meat or meat substitutes	150 calories per serving	3 ounces fish, chicken, or turkey (without the skin) or lean beef 1/2 cup beans 1/2 cup tofu 2 tablespoons peanut butter 1/4 cup unsalted nuts 3 tablespoons seeds 2 eggs
Dairy products	90 calories per serving	1 cup skim or 1% milk 1 cup nonfat or light soy milk 1 cup nonfat yogurt 1 ounce cheese 1/4 cup low-fat cheese 1/2 cup nonfat or low-fat cottage cheese

Fats	45 calories per serving	1 teaspoon oil or butter
		2 tablespoons or 1/8 avocado
		2 tablespoons hummus
		1 tablespoon low-fat mayonnaise
		1 tablespoon salad dressing
		2 tablespoons reduced-calorie salad dressing
		1 tablespoon cream
		2 tablespoons half-and-half
		1 tablespoon sour cream
		2 tablespoons nonfat sour cream
		1 tablespoon cream cheese
		2 tablespoons nonfat cream cheese
Sweets and treats	80 calories per serving	1/2 cup nonfat frozen yogurt
		1 ounce candy
		4 ounces wine
		12 ounces light beer

Total number of servings: Grains____ Fruits____ Vegetables____ Meat or Meat Substitutes____
Dairy Products____ Fats____ Sweets and Treats____ Calories____

For long-term success, you should get into the habit of comparing your hand with the food you are eating. In general, the volume of a fist is about one cup and the volume of the palm of your hand is about a half cup. The palm of your hand is also generally equivalent to a three-ounce portion of meat. The volume of your thumb is about one tablespoon, while the tip of your thumb is about one teaspoon. For the first couple of weeks, use a measuring cup and a scale to make sure you are estimating correctly, but as time goes on and you feel more comfortable with serving sizes, you can just use your hand.

Some people find it helpful to compare food sizes with common objects. One cup is equal to a tennis ball. A half cup is the size of a deck of cards. A three-ounce portion of meat is also the size of a deck of cards. One-quarter cup is about the size of a golf ball. One ounce of nuts is also about the size of a golf ball. One tablespoon is about the size of a matchbox.

In the Personal Nutrition Plan, you'll see that everything is kept quite simple. You want simplicity so that it will be easy to follow. Each food serving has a certain number of calories associated with it, but some foods will be a little over or a little under. That's okay; it all evens out. Also, a serving size does not mean the same thing as a portion size. Portion sizes at a meal typically consist of one, two, or three serving sizes of any one food category. The table indicates the size of one serving, but that doesn't mean that you can have only one serving of a food group at each meal.

Finally, you need to know what to do if you have anything from the Sweets and Treats category. Of course, you're going to try to minimize this category, but there will be times when you just can't resist. Perhaps you want a small glass of wine with dinner, or maybe it's your birthday and you want to enjoy a piece of birthday cake. That's fine. Here's how you account for it. Each sweet serving is considered to be 80 calories. It would need to be counted in the grains category, so you would simply reduce the appropriate number of servings in that category for that day. This grain category is logical to reduce from because the group is largely carbohydrate-based. The big difference with Sweets and Treats is that these foods are made primarily of refined carbohydrates rather than whole-grain, complex carbohydrates, and they also usually contain quite a bit of fat.

For the first two weeks, avoid Sweets and Treats altogether. After that, I suggest you limit Sweets and Treats to one serving a day. Each serving is about 80 calories and does not contain many valuable nutrients, but in small amounts, these kinds of foods can easily fit into your Personal Nutrition Plan. Choose a low-calorie option when possible. In order to balance your calories for the day, make sure you deduct one serving from the grain group for every Sweets and Treats serving (i.e., 1 sweet = 1 grain equivalent).

If you go over your serving allotments for a day, don't treat it like a catastrophe. Just get back on track and keep going. Remember, this isn't about needing to be perfect.

If you are someone who does best with more of a structure, you can follow the plan below for the first two weeks and stick to those foods that are listed in the Serving Sizes at a Glance chart on page 73. The following is an example of the Personal Nutrition Plan: 1,400 calories. You can add or subtract food servings if your plan is higher or lower in calories.

BREAKFAST: 2 GRAINS, 1 FRUIT, 1 DAIRY

EXAMPLE: 1 toasted whole-wheat English muffin, 1 cup fruit blended with 1 cup nonfat yogurt in a blender.

LUNCH: 2 VEGETABLES, 1 MEAT, 1 FRUIT, 2 FAT, 2 GRAINS

EXAMPLE: Large green salad with mixed raw vegetables and 3 ounces chicken, sprinkled with cranberry raisins and 1 tablespoon salad dressing, 1 whole-wheat roll, 1 teaspoon butter substitute.

4 P.M. SNACK: 1 FRUIT, 1 DAIRY

EXAMPLE: 1 orange, 1 string cheese stick.

DINNER: 1 MEAT, 2 GRAINS, 2 VEGETABLES, 1 FAT

EXAMPLE: 3 ounces fish, 1 cup brown rice, 1 cup cooked vegetables sautéed in 1 teaspoon olive oil.

There will always be some foods you aren't sure how to count. The best way to figure it out is to think of the separate main ingredients that are in the food and assign the food to a food group. Don't make it more difficult than it needs to be. If you are watching portion sizes, you will do fine. For the first two weeks, stick with the foods that are easy to classify and listed in the Serving Sizes at a Glance chart. This will give you time to get used to the system.

An important point to remember is that if you feel hungry (true hunger) on your plan or get lightheaded, add a snack. In general, I recommend having a 4 P.M. snack every day, because this will prevent you from going to dinner too hungry and potentially overeating. Feel free to add extra vegetables or fruit. You can actually have as many vegetables as you want, as long as they are not starchy vegetables such as corn and potatoes (starchy vegetables are considered grains). If that doesn't help, have an extra piece of low-fat cheese or a small amount of hummus. That should give you enough extra fuel to make it to your next meal.

Variation of the Personal Nutrition Plan

If counting servings of food groups drives you crazy, you can simplify your eating plan by learning a few basic guidelines for creating portion-controlled, healthful meals.

FOR BREAKFAST

Fill a six-inch bowl with one grain, dairy product (or meat or meat substitute), and fruit. Some examples are:

Unsweetened cereal with nonfat milk and fruit

Unflavored cooked oatmeal with nonfat milk, sprinkled with raisins or dried cranberries

Nonfat yogurt and fresh fruit sprinkled with wheat germ, low-fat granola, or Grape-Nuts

Low-fat cottage cheese with fruit and a slice of whole-wheat toast

Scrambled eggs with mixed vegetables and a couple of tablespoons of low-fat shredded cheese with a slice of whole-wheat toast

FOR LUNCH AND DINNER

Fill one quarter of a ten-inch plate with grains (equivalent to about 1 cup or 2 grain servings), one quarter of the plate with meat or meat substitute (equivalent to about 1 serving of meat or meat substitute), and half the plate with fruits and vegetables (equivalent to 2 to 3 servings of fruits and vegetables).

If you are trying to lose weight and it is not happening, it is almost always due to one of three reasons:

- Your portion sizes are larger than they should be.

- You don't realize that certain high-calorie foods have been slipped into the preparation process. (This often happens when you eat out at restaurants, where fats are used more liberally.)

- You are unconsciously eating food during the day (nibbling a little here and there), and you are not counting it. All of it counts.

After adjusting for the points above, if you are still not losing weight, consider cutting back on the number of fat servings in your plan. Fat is often slipped into prepared foods, so you usually don't have to go out of your way to get your daily fat servings. Although the good thing about fat is that it keeps us feeling full longer, remember that it has more than twice the number of calories per gram of carbohydrate and protein. So even in small amounts the calories in fat add up quickly.

Counting Calories

If you prefer to count calories instead of food serving sizes, that's fine. You will probably want to purchase a calorie-counting book. I particularly like Corinne T. Netzer's *The Complete Book of Food Counts.* Even if you are counting calories, it is still important for you to have a balanced diet. In general, people typically get enough grains, fat, and protein, but they struggle to eat enough fruits and vegetables, so track your fruit and vegetable intake; otherwise concentrate on total calories. If you think you may not be meeting your dairy needs, take a daily calcium supplement.

Finally, remember that any good nutrition plan does not rest on your food intake alone but should be paired with an increase in your daily activity level as well. Exercise matters!

FITNESS: CREATING YOUR PERSONAL FITNESS PLAN

This week I'd like you to design your own personal fitness program. I want you to make it simple enough that you can follow the overall layout of the plan forever. At no time in your life does exercise become less important, so don't make exercise so labor-intensive or impractical that you can't or won't want to do it on a long-term basis. The activities you choose may be varied so that you don't get bored, but the basic plan will stay roughly the same.

When you design your own personal fitness program, you need to think about the three basic components: *cardiorespiratory, strength,* and *flexibility.* The Basic Fitness Plan below incorporates all of these basic components to keep you healthy no matter what your age. I don't expect you to jump right in and do all of it right away. You will work up to it slowly, but this will give you an idea of the overall plan you should shoot for.

Basic Fitness Plan

Cardiovascular Activity (increases fitness level)

- Walk at a brisk pace or do some other moderate-intensity aerobic exercise every day for 30 minutes.

- Eventually, add on 20 to 30 minutes of higher-intensity aerobic exercise three times a week.

Resistance (increases strength)

- Do 15 minutes of resistance exercises two to three times a week on nonconsecutive days.

- If you want to increase your muscle mass, you can increase the duration, frequency, and resistance.

STRETCHING (INCREASES FLEXIBILITY)

- Stretch for at least 5 minutes every day.

- For added benefit, you can increase the duration of the stretching period.

For cardiorespiratory or aerobic activity, you don't need to do anything fancier than just walking. But you do need to do something you enjoy; otherwise you won't keep it up. Choose any aerobic activity you like. Options include walking or running, bicycling, swimming, dancing, jumping on a trampoline, skipping rope, rowing, cross-country skiing—anything that makes you move constantly over a 30- to 60-minute period. Aerobic exercise should be the foundation of your exercise program. I suggest you start by walking a half hour every day at a moderately brisk pace. Eventually, you should add 20 to 30 minutes three times a week, increasing the intensity of your exercise. A brisk walk at three to four miles per hour takes your heart rate to 50 percent of your maximum. When you step it up in intensity for the additional 20 to 30 minutes three times a week, you should work to achieve a heart rate of 60 to 80 percent of your maximum heart rate during that additional time period. You can easily determine what your maximum heart rate should be by using this formula:

> **Maximum heart rate = 220 - your age**

This number is the maximum beats per minute your heart should pump. You can count the beats over a 15-second period (on your neck beside the Adam's apple area or along your wrist next to the thumb) and multiply by four to get the number of beats per minute. Now here's a disclaimer: this formula gives a number that is only an estimate and can vary by up to 20 beats. Also, your maximum heart rate by this formula doesn't tell you anything about the shape you are in; it is simply a rough gauge of how much work you should push your heart to do based on your age. You don't need to push yourself to your maximum heart rate, nor is it recommended. To achieve higher cardiorespiratory fitness, you want to get your heart rate to 60 to 80 percent of your maximum for at least 20 to 30 minutes three times a week. But remember, any activity is better than none, so please do not get too caught up in the numbers. If you never checked your heart rate over your entire life but just walked for exercise every day, you would be just fine!

Estimate your personal maximum heart rate by the equation:
Maximum heart rate = 220 - age = ____ beats per minute
50% of maximum heart rate = (.5 x max heart rate) = ____ beats per minute
60% of maximum heart rate = (.6 x max heart rate) = ____ beats per minute
80% of maximum heart rate = (.8 x max heart rate) = ____ beats per minute

---

Certainly you can do any cardio exercise—you don't have to walk. Mix it up with different aerobic activities to cross-train different muscle groups. If you choose walking, consider purchasing a pedometer, which is an easy way of recording your daily steps taken. Your goal is to take 10,000 steps a day, which is about four miles. I particularly like the Omron HJ-112 pedometer, which records your steps even if you place the pedometer in your pocket or purse. It also has a convenient memory feature.

Resistance exercises work your muscles so they get stronger. To strengthen and tone your muscles, you need to do these exercises for at least 15 minutes twice a week. That's not so bad! You really don't have to do the resistance exercises much at all to start to see benefits. If you want to build muscle and bulk up, you will need to increase the frequency and intensity of the workout. Remember not to stress the same muscle groups on two consecutive days. It takes at least twenty-four hours for muscle groups to repair themselves after they have been stressed. In Week 5 we'll go over a simple at-home routine you can do, but feel free to read ahead if you want to get started now.

Flexibility exercises should be done every day for about 5 minutes. Do them when you are warm, after your walking or other cardio exercise. No special equipment is necessary. We'll go over a flexibility routine in Week 7, but you can start now if you like!

Don't worry, you aren't expected to jump in and do everything right now. You'll work up to it gradually. Also, I think you'll be surprised at how easy and routine this will become once you get going. You will also start to feel the difference quite quickly in your body, energy, attention, and mood. Exercise is really pretty amazing if you think about it. If someone created a pill that could actually provide all the wonderful physical and mental benefits that exercise offers, you can bet that people everywhere would be popping those pills as if there were no tomorrow. But then, no pill like this exists *and* if you did it that way, you wouldn't be able to feel quite so proud of yourself for feeling so good. Also, exercise is free!

Last week I asked you to just start moving every day. This week I'd like you to try to consistently get in 30 minutes (on average) of some type of aerobic exercise every day. Perhaps you want to do 45 minutes only five days a week because there are two days each week when you start at work too early. That's okay. Just aim for 30 minutes a day on average of some form of physical activity. Walking is the most common activity, but it is by no means the only thing you can do. Do what you like to do. Make it fun. Listen to music or socialize with a buddy. If you find it fun, you'll keep doing it. If you find it drudgery, you won't, so it's important to personalize this physical activity so that you enjoy it.

LEARN IT!

- You are more likely to succeed in your goals if you know how to be your own best coach.

- Your BMI should be less than 25 for optimal health.

- To lose one pound of fat (not water weight), you must accumulate a deficit of 3,500 calories.

- To maintain your current weight, your daily calories should be roughly equal to your weight (in pounds) x 11.

- An optimal exercise program should consist of:

  - 30 minutes of moderate-intensity aerobic exercise most days of the week with 20 minutes of additional higher-intensity aerobic exercise three days of the week

  - 15 minutes of resistance exercises two to three times a week

  - Flexibility exercises daily for 5 minutes or longer if needed

- Maximum heart rate = 220 - your age.

PERSONALIZE IT!

This week, work on your Resistant Brain.

Although your brain can change, it is generally set up to resist change, especially sudden change. People who are successful in initiating and maintaining major behavioral changes usually make them one step a time.

Here are some examples of how people in The Program have personalized this brain principle and put it into action.

- Karen W., a 64-year-old, wanted to lose 10 pounds, but she did not want to follow a structured diet or feel hungry. She decided to simply cut out desserts until she reached her goal. It took her seven months, and although there were times she wished she was losing faster, she ultimately reached her goal and never felt significantly deprived.

- Peter M., a 39-year-old banker, changed only what he ate for lunch. He decided to have a turkey sandwich, fruit, and a diet drink for lunch every day instead of his usual cheeseburger, milk shake, and fries. He lost 24 pounds in twelve weeks with just that one change. Small changes can indeed result in big outcomes!

- Harry R., a 66-year-old retired radiologist, was not a big fan of exercise. To get started, he began walking on his home treadmill during TV commercials at night. Every day he increased the time by just one minute such that he worked his way up to 60 minutes over two months. Then he began to run, sometimes running 30 minutes and sometimes 60. He ran his first 10k race six months after starting this workout regimen. Although adding just one minute of exercise time each day seemed silly to him at first, he ultimately became more physically fit than he had ever been in his life and was able to sustain it for years afterward.

LIVE IT!

- Review last week's goals and create this week's short-term goals. Work toward your long-term goals gradually.

- Pick your Personal Nutrition Plan.

- Learn how to estimate food servings.

- Make sure you eat breakfast every morning.

- Aim for 30 minutes of moderately intense exercise each day.

MASTERING STRESS

Change your thoughts and you change your world.

–NORMAN VINCENT PEALE

STRESS. WHAT IS IT? You know it when you feel it, and these days you may be feeling it a lot. It's that knot in your stomach when you are stuck in traffic and your meeting started fifteen minutes ago, or that tightness you get in your neck when you have been working all day to meet deadlines and you have eight people coming over for dinner. Too many obligations, too many pressures, too little time to step back and simply enjoy the moment.

You can't talk about making positive changes in your health without addressing the topic of stress. In fact, stress management is one of the most important skill you need for staying healthy in the fast-paced world we live in today. I'm not suggesting our lives are more stressful now than they were in the past, but I do think our modern world comes with its own unique set of stressors. Technology has improved our lives in many ways, but it has also created a brand-new set of stresses such as those associated with multitasking, information overload, and heightened expectations about what we can reasonably accomplish. Humans also have a special physiology that makes stress particularly tricky. Did you know that humans, unlike any other animal, can actually turn on the stress response just by *thinking* of something stressful? All other animals require sensory input (through smell, sound, sight, or touch) before the alarm bells sound. We humans, though, can think our way into stress even if nothing stressful is happening.

Stress, then, is the physiologic response to an event. It is not the event itself. This is an important concept to understand because although you may not be able to prevent external stress-producing events from happening, you can learn to control your response to those events. You can influence the way thought patterns work in your brain, and you can learn to use this fact to your advantage in a big way.

Let's go over how your brain is set up. It can be broken down into three evolutionarily distinct parts: reptilian, mammalian, and human.

There's the **brainstem,** which is reptilian in its evolutionary development. It is a tubular structure at the base of your brain that attaches to your spinal cord. Your brainstem is involved in the basic functions of living, such as your breathing and your heartbeat.

Above the reptilian part lies the mammalian brain, the home of the emotional **limbic system.** It is here that the stress response originates in your **amygdala** (a-MIG-duh-la), and it is also here that memory formation occurs—specifically

MODEL FOR BRAIN EVOLUTION

Human — Cerebral Cortex

Limbic System

Brainstem

Mammalian —

Reptilian —

in your **hippocampus.** The amygdala (emotion) and hippocampus (memory) sit side by side and talk to each other. Given their close connection, it should come as no surprise that the strongest memories have strong emotions attached to them.

Finally, there is the **cerebral cortex,** the most evolutionarily developed district of your brain, which separates humans from other animals. The cerebral cortex is what defines the human experience. It makes up the outer layer of your brain and encases your inner core limbic system. The cerebral cortex, particularly the frontal cortex, is where you analyze information, solve problems, and create.

Let's discuss the stress response. All animals have a physiologic stress response, and it is beautifully choreographed to do one main thing: keep you alive. It works like this. Let's imagine you are out on the savanna hunting for food. Suddenly you see a lion, and he's ready to pounce on you. The visual stimulus of the lion travels to the "input center" in the core of your brain, the **thalamus,** which is shaped like a tiny football. The thalamus is the receiving station for all information from your senses. The thalamus rushes this information over to the amygdala in record time. The thalamus also sends the information to the cerebral cortex in the outermost brain, though it sends it a bit more slowly. The amygdala's job is to quickly scan the incoming information and compare it to past experiences you have had. This scanning system allows your amygdala to determine, in a fraction of a second, whether the incoming information signals danger. If it does (or if your amygdala simply thinks it does), it will fire up the "stress response."

Anxiety Disorders are the most common type of psychiatric disorder in the United States. About 40 million people experience them.

But I want to point out that your brain is not perfect. Your amygdala will sometimes mismatch information and fire the stress response falsely. The incoming information may not be life-threatening at all—but it may have enough similarities to a past traumatic event that the stress response will fire anyway. You also have primitive behavioral circuitry that has evolved over millions of years and is more or less "hardwired" into your brain. The stress response can therefore fire if your brain interprets incoming information in ways you find innately threatening, such as abandonment, rejection, or loss of control, or when you find yourself in a new or unfamiliar situation. It's this last one that makes it difficult for the brain when it comes to adopting new behavior.

Since the information coming in from the thalamus reaches the amygdala faster than it reaches the cerebral cortex, you sometimes have a visceral response to an event before you can even figure out why you feel the way you do. Let's say you are hiking on a trail, and all of a sudden, in the middle of the trail you see a long, brown ropy-looking object. Your heart will race and your muscles will tighten reflexively because the image of what you just saw has been quickly scanned by your amygdala and it reads, "Danger! Snake!" This information quickly reaches your cerebral cortex, which then processes the information and sends a message back to the amygdala, saying, "No, no, we've processed this image up here and it looks like a stick. It's not a snake. You can relax." So, the amygdala turns off and you eventually start breathing easier. The same type of response can happen when you are going through your incoming e-mails and you see the name of someone who often sends you e-mails with bad news.

When the stress response fires, the sympathetic nervous system springs into action. The sympathetic nervous system is one of two branches of the autonomic nervous system, also known as the involuntary nervous system. The sympathetic system generally speeds things up, and the parasympathetic system generally slows things down. You can think of the sympathetic system like the gas pedal in your car and the parasympathetic nervous system like the brakes. It's the sympathetic system that gets called into action during the stress response. Your adrenal glands also get into the act. These glands sit on top of your kidneys, and when they are activated, they pump out epinephrine and cortisol. Epinephrine is also known as adrenaline, and cortisol is often referred to as "the stress chemical."

Your body responds to the heightened sympathetic and adrenal gland activity in the following ways:

- **Your heart rate increases.** This allows your heart to pump more blood to your muscles and organs, thereby bringing in fresh supplies of oxygen and glucose.

- **Your breathing quickens** to increase the amount of oxygen your lungs absorb.

- **Your blood pressure elevates** to make sure all of the organs in your body, including your brain, are infused with vital nutrients such as oxygen and glucose.

- **Blood flow diverts from your gut to your skeletal muscles,** preparing you for "fight or flight." The performance of your muscles is critical in the stress response because your muscles determine how fast you can run and how hard you can fight.

- **Blood flow shifts in the brain** away from the higher cerebral cortex to the lower, more primitive areas. This allows for heightened sensory perception and quicker reaction times, but the shift in blood flow reduces your ability to solve complex problems.

- **Your libido decreases.** Nature has decided that when there is a life-threatening event, it is not a good time to reproduce.

- **Your digestion turns off.** Your gut largely shuts down during the stress response because your body has more important things to do. Your body's focus is on keeping you alive; it can process what you ate for lunch later.

- **The muscles around your lower back, neck, and jaw tighten.** You can't have a floppy spine or jaw if you want to run fast or fight well.

- **Your blood sugar increases.** This is important because your muscles and brain need more fuel.

- **Fats are released into your bloodstream.** Both fats and sugars can be used as fuel for your muscles as you fight or run away from danger, although sugar is the preferred fuel.

- **Circulating platelets in your blood activate** so that if you get cut during the fight-or-flight response the bleeding will stop more readily.

- **You sweat,** to help your body cool down quickly.

The stress response, as you can see, is a beautifully coordinated set of reactions designed to keep you alive during a life-threatening event. Stress is not necessarily bad for your health; it can even be beneficial, but only if it occurs *occasionally* and *briefly.* It is meant to be a short-term response. Once the danger is over, the stress response is supposed to stop. In animals other than humans, it does stop. If you were a mouse running from a cat, you would run into a hole, and when you didn't see, hear, or smell the cat anymore, your stress response would turn off. Humans, however, have a highly developed cerebral cortex that allows the processing of complex

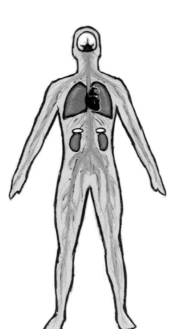

- Blood flow shifts away from cerebral cortex

- Breathing quickens

- Blood sugar increases

- Circulating fat increases

- Platelets activate

- Sexual libido lowers

- Spine muscles tighten

- Heart rate increases

- Blood pressure elevates

- Blood flow diverts from gut to muscles

- Sweating occurs

thoughts, so you, the human, would stay in that hole and even though you didn't see, hear, or smell the cat, your mind would still be racing along, planning how you could escape. In other words, your highly developed cerebral cortex has—and I want you to understand this—*a direct route to the amygdala.* You can activate the stress response directly from thoughts generated by your cerebral cortex. You don't need a real event to fire the stress response. You can just think yourself into stress. So for most people, the amygdala fires many times a day just because of what they are thinking and not because of any life-threatening situations.

Chronic Stress *can actually damage the hippocampus and lead to memory impairment.*

What does this have to do with your health? Everything! Chronic stimulation of the stress response affects your health in a striking number of ways, so having a handle on the stress response is critical for maintaining a healthy life. When stress continues unchecked, your body starts to display:

- **High blood pressure.** High blood pressure is damaging to the inner lining of your blood vessels, creating nicks and ultimately allowing the formation of cholesterol plaques to clog your arteries.

- **High blood sugar level.** A high blood sugar level is also damaging to the inner lining of the blood vessels, accelerating the formation of arterial plaques. This is because blood sugar attaches to proteins on the artery's inner lining, and this ultimately initiates an inflammatory process. People with high blood sugar (seen in uncontrolled diabetes) experience higher incidences of heart attacks, strokes, nerve problems, and infections. A high blood sugar level makes sense in the short term if you are in a life-threatening situation, but your body is not designed to experience this on a chronic basis.

- **High cholesterol level.** Cholesterol is not often discussed as a consequence of stress, but in fact LDL (bad) cholesterol does go up during stress. Studies in medical students have demonstrated that LDL levels shoot up right before these students take exams.

- **Increased frequency of heart attacks and strokes.** Chronic stress damages the inner lining of the arteries by creating higher levels of blood sugar, blood pressure, and cholesterol, which promote plaque formation. In addition, stress increases the stickiness of your platelets, making your blood more likely to clot. Plaque in the arteries plus sticky platelets equals a dangerous combination for your blood vessels, resulting in heart attacks and strokes.

- **Increased heart arrhythmias.** Your heart is more likely to have an irregular rhythm when the sympathetic system is going full tilt and your heart cells are bathing in epinephrine.

- **Increased infections.** Your immune cells keep infections and cancers in check, but they themselves are suppressed when you are under stress. In the stress response, your body is designed to channel all of its energy into running away or fighting. Daily maintenance activities are put on the back burner, so wound healing and cancer surveillance are given a lower priority. This is fine if the stress is real and short-lived, but not if it simmers unabated.

- **Decreased mental acuity.** Blood flow shifts away from your higher cortical areas during stress, so although you may have heightened senses and a heightened reaction time, you are less able to think rationally and clearly. The stress chemical, cortisol, is also toxic in high levels to your neurons. If you sprinkle cortisol on neurons in a lab Petri dish, they shrivel up and die. The neurons in your hippocampus are especially full of cortisol receptors, so this area of your brain can actually shrink when you are subjected to severe, ongoing stress.

- **Headaches, temporomandibular pain, neck pain, and lower-back pain.** The muscles around your spine and jaw tighten with stress to prepare you better for running or fighting. This muscle tightening is designed to be short term, though. See the box on page 103 for a complete description of the three major types of headaches.

- **Irritable bowel symptoms.** Because the gastrointestinal (GI) system is controlled by the sympathetic and parasympathetic nerve systems, the GI tract is particularly sensitive to stress, manifesting as diarrhea, constipation, bloating, or abdominal pain.

- **Depression.** As we will discuss at length in Week 8, your mood is tightly connected to the same pathways as the stress response. Stress can lead to depression, and depression itself is a form of stress.

- **Fatigue.** Most people find emotional stress far more fatiguing than physical stress. In stress, energy is diverted in preparation for fight or flight, so there isn't much energy left over for anything else.

- **Sleep disruption.** In order to relax and fall asleep, the sympathetic nervous system must be calmed and the parasympathetic nervous system must be activated. The same tricks that work for reducing stress also work for encouraging sleep (see page 100).

- **Increased perception of pain.** When the brain and body are subjected to ongoing, chronic stress, there are shifts in several of the chemicals in both the brain and body that control pain perception. For example, in chronic stress or depression, pain syndromes worsen. Serotonin levels are often found to be lower in both depression and chronic pain, and elevation of serotonin levels can help in pain control. Also, chronic pain itself is considered a stress that can lead to depression, while chronic stress or depression can lead to a pain syndrome. It is important to treat pain when trying to lower depression or stress, and it is important to treat depression and stress when trying to lower pain.

- **Gastroesophageal reflux disease (GERD) or heartburn.** This is seen in chronic stress due to decreased gut motility and increased stomach acid.

- **Weight changes.** Weight loss or weight gain can be a consequence of stress. In really life-threatening events, your gut motility shuts down. This makes sense. Why would your body be designed to stop and graze when a lion is about to pounce on you? If you do eat during acute, high-stress times, you may even vomit due to this gut shutdown; food simply does not move through. Emotional eating is typically a response to lower but chronic stress; we will discuss the physiology behind this in Week 9.

- **Decreased performance.** In acute stress, there is initially an increase in both mental and physical performance, but in chronic stress, performance declines.

- **Faster aging.** Yes, stress can age you faster and shorten your life. Your chromosomes (which sit at the command and control center within each of your cells) have protective caps on each of their ends called *telomeres*. With aging, the telomere caps wear down, and once the caps have completely worn down, the cell dies. Stress wears these caps down more quickly and is felt to speed up the aging process by as much as ten to fifteen years. Stress also decreases neurogenesis, the production of new brain cells. So, in addition to aging, stress can also worsen memory and lower the ability to learn new information.

So you see what I mean about the dangers of stress? Clearly it is important to know how to keep your stress in check. I want to point out again, though, that small amounts of stress can be actually good for you. Not only can it improve your mental and physical performance (again, we're talking about *short-term stress*), it can also help your brain physically restructure itself, so that it can become more powerful and resilient.

Your brain is really like a muscle. You need to push a muscle and even tear it a little in order to make it stronger. When you stress a muscle, it comes back saying "Wow, I wasn't prepared for that. I'm going to grow back even stronger so I can handle things better next time." And then it physically changes so it can handle stress better the next time, growing back with thicker muscle fibers. The same thing happens in your brain. Your brain reconfigures its networks and tightens its synapses, so after a short-term stress response, it comes back stronger and more resilient.

The lesson here is: don't be afraid of short-lived stress. In fact, it's okay if you even thrive on it. Some people do. Don't hesitate to challenge yourself. You'll grow stronger in the process. But here's the catch: the stress that comes with those challenges must be enjoyed by you and/or must be of short duration. You need to be able to turn off the stress response when you want to, and this is where you need to start thinking about strategies for stress control. You need to be in charge of your stress response so that it works *for* you and not *against* you.

In fact, if there is one message you should hear in all of this, it is this: it is not necessarily how much stress people have in their lives, it is how they feel about it and whether they are able to shut off the stress response when they want to so that it does not simmer unchecked. Learning how to control the stress response is perhaps the most important lesson you can learn when it comes to good health. Trust me on this. There is almost nothing you can do for yourself that is more important than developing solid strategies to deal with stress.

If you're like most people, you may be reading this and thinking "Sure, I have some stress, but who doesn't? How would I know if my stress levels are high enough to be hurting me?" Unfortunately, there isn't a quantitative test to check to see if your stress levels are hurting your health, but there is one way you can tell. Think about how you feel when you are in a very stressful situation. Identify that feeling.

How often do you get that feeling? Most people can define when their stress feels good (as in excitement) and when it feels bad (as in fear). You might be the type of person who thrives on stress. It feels good to you; you find it exhilarating. But what if it starts to feel bad and you start feeling anxious? Can you turn it off? If the answer is yes, you are fine. If the answer is no, you have some work to do.

Long-term Strategies to Reduce Stress

How can you turn off the stress response and keep it off? It's probably easiest to divide the strategies into short-term and long-term. Long-term strategies help you prevent unnecessary activation of the stress response in the first place. Short-term strategies help you turn off the stress response when it is active, but you no longer want it to be.

One of the best long-term and short-term strategies for stress control is to maintain a regular exercise program. I know, you've heard this before, but it is really true. When you exercise regularly, you raise the threshold for the release of the stress response. You not only become much more relaxed immediately after exercise, you also find that your stress response will simply not fire as readily. How does that happen? It's an amazing process.

First, when you exercise, your heart rate increases, and this stimulates your heart to release a hormone called atrial natriuretic peptide. This hormone then crosses the blood–brain barrier of your brain, goes right over to your emotional limbic system, and turns off the stress response. See what I mean about amazing?

Your brain also produces endorphins, which work like morphine; endocannabinoids, (which work like marijuana); serotonin, a feel-good, calming neurotransmitter; dopamine, a feel-good, motivating neurotransmitter; and brain-derived neurotrophic factor (BDNF), which fertilizes your brain cells somewhat like Miracle-Gro does plants. Your moving muscles also release growth factors that stimulate the production of proteins used to lay down the infrastructure for new nerve networks, and tighten the already existing nerve connections, making it easier for you to learn, pay attention, and stay happy—while also being calm and relaxed. Wow! It's almost too easy, right?

In addition to regular exercise, you need to eat regular meals. Your body is designed to eat about every four hours while you are awake, and when you don't, the stress response fires. You don't need to eat much at any one time, but you should have something about every four hours. It's also best to choose foods that keep your blood sugar levels nice and steady until your next meal. If you eat in a way that causes your blood sugar level to spike and then plummet, your stress response will often fire.

Your body is designed to get an average of eight hours of sleep per night. You may need a little more or a little less, but if you try to get by on less sleep than your body needs, the stress response activates. It should therefore come as no surprise that the health consequences we see in people who are chronically sleep-deprived are exactly the same health consequences we see in people who are chronically stressed.

You need to learn how to slow down and enjoy more of less. This is another long-term stress management skill. We live in a fast-paced world, and overscheduling ourselves has become the norm. You are not designed to be on the go 24/7. Stop and figure out what is really important to you. Decide what you absolutely need to be happy and what is negotiable. Then prioritize your schedule. You don't have to say yes to every project that comes along at work or go to every party you are invited to. Slow down. Smell the flowers. Try to spend more time doing fewer things but enjoying them more. It's your life, your one life. Live it the way that makes you the happiest.

Set aside time each day to nurture yourself and relax. Just as you can't drive your car without stopping to refuel every now and then, so it is with your mind and body. Go for a walk, read a book, take a warm bath, listen to a rerun of *Friends* while you're making dinner, or spend time with a buddy while you exercise. You can weave in some time for yourself if you are creative. Take time to "refuel your tank" on a regular basis, and you will end up with much more energy and much less stress in the long run.

Create a supportive social network. Studies show that having positive relationships with friends and family leads to not just a higher quality of life but a longer life as well. In fact, the "fight-or-flight" stress response is not the only survival mechanism we have evolved for survival. Women, in particular, probably because of their physical limitations of size and strength, have evolved what has been labeled the "tend-and-befriend" survival coping mechanism. We humans are wired for social connection, and it makes sense that surrounding ourselves with a sympathetic community evolved, at least partially, as a survival mechanism. Recent research has focused on mirror neurons in the brain that enable humans to have a tremendous amount of empathy for one another. We are designed to cooperate as well as learn from one another. During positive social interactions, the brain produces higher levels of dopamine, oxytocin, and serotonin, the feel-good chemicals that help us stay happy and calm.

Meditation and yoga can also be effective for controlling stress by allowing you to tap into the autonomic, "involuntary" nervous system. There are two nerve networks that weave themselves throughout the body: the voluntary nerves and the involuntary nerves. Your voluntary system is the one you control easily. If you want to lift your hand, you can willingly fire the nerves that activate the muscles that move your hand. The second nerve network is the involuntary system, made up of the sympathetic and parasympathetic nerves that I described earlier. This system is harder to control, but with practice you can learn how to influence it. Although the sympathetic and parasympathetic systems are considered "involuntary," the truth is that you can actually learn how to activate them, and you can become really quite good at it. For example, you can activate your sympathetic system by thinking of something that excites you. It can be something that makes you happy, such as a concert you are about to attend, or it can be something you are stressing about, such as a deadline for a paper. If you want to turn the sympathetic system off, you can do slow deep breathing or focus on a scene or a thought that you find calming and peaceful. When you do meditation or yoga, the deep breathing and focus of these activities activate the parasympathetic system.

Let me be quick to say that learning how to manage stress is not all about learning to be mellow. You can be incredibly vital, energetic, and productive without having your stress response firing all the time. What you need is a balance between the sympathetic and parasympathetic nerve systems. Just as you shouldn't step on the gas pedal and the brake of your car at the same time, so must you learn how to share the power within the autonomic nervous system.

There are four possible outcomes when talking about the balance between the sympathetic and parasympathetic systems. You can be healthy-sympathetic-dominant, where you feel energetic and challenged, as, for example, when you are getting ready to go onstage to play the lead in *Hamlet* or run a fifty-yard dash. Or you may be unhealthy-sympathetic-dominant and feel frazzled and anxious in these same situations. Likewise, you may be healthy-parasympathetic-dominant while relaxing on a blanket at the beach or drifting off to sleep. Or you can be unhealthy-parasympathetic-dominant, and experience lethargy, apathy, and depression.

Your thoughts are also crucial in winning the battle of stress. Studies show that people who focus on the positive aspects of their lives (what is going right and what they are grateful for) have lower stress levels than those who focus on the negative. Simply switching your thoughts from negative to positive (such as thinking of something that brings you great joy) shifts your brain and body's physiology into a healthier mode. Of course you can use this as a quick, short-term method of turning off stress, but maintaining a positive outlook in general, which is something you can practice and improve in, is an excellent long-term strategy for stress management. It also helps to learn more about why you have certain feelings or responses. Knowing what pushes your buttons and why you respond the way you do is a pivotal part of maturing. You can use this knowledge to change the way you feel and respond. This strategy engages your sophisticated, higher-functioning, cerebral cortex and is referred to as cognitive restructuring.

Your general outlook and way of thinking influence how active your stress response is. As I mentioned before, thoughts or incoming information can trigger the stress response if the amygdala interprets them as threatening. Mismatches in this process, as I've said before, can fire the stress response. Having a better understanding of what pushes your buttons and why you respond the way you do can reduce the number of mismatches and therefore lower your stress long term. This isn't frivolous, new-age kind of talk. This is about physically restructuring your nerve networks. Your cerebral cortex and your more primitive, emotional limbic system (where your amygdala lives) are tightly connected. You can head off amygdala activity by sending in nerve activity from your higher-functioning cerebral cortex. Jim may think, for example, "Okay, Molly was a little rude when she spoke to me, but she has been under a lot of stress and it doesn't mean she doesn't love me anymore and that all of a sudden she is just going to walk away from the relationship. She's worried about losing her job. I know that when I feel threatened with rejection I often lash out at her, but I'm not going to do that this time. I'm going to take the high road here and let it go. I know Molly loves me. We have a great relationship, and I'm going to tell her how much I appreciate her." There, you talked yourself out of the stress response, and every time you think this way, your neural synapses cement together more strongly and new nerve networks develop. The more you repeat this kind of thinking, the easier it is to think this way the next time a similar situation comes up. Your brain changes *physically* in response to your thoughts.

Short-term Strategies to Reduce Stress

Short-term strategies for stress reduction are important, too. Let's say you have incorporated several long-term stress reduction measures into your life; there are still going to be times when you feel the stress response start to fire. What short-term techniques can you employ to turn the stress response off?

First, recognize the way your body feels when it is stressed. Does your jaw tighten? Does your neck hurt? Do you feel a knot in your stomach? Do you feel you have to escape? The easiest and quickest way to turn off the stress response is to do slow, deep breathing. You can turn off the stress response physiologically in less than 60 seconds with a few, very slow deep breaths. Here's what you do: Count to five slowly while inhaling, hold for five counts, and then exhale for five counts. After five or so breaths, focus on what it is you are truly thankful for. Picture it in your mind, and really concentrate on this feeling. You can think any pleasant thought you want to turn off the stress response, but *feelings of gratitude turn out to be the most effective.*

The deep breathing sends negative feedback to your brain, reassuring it that you are not in the middle of a life-threatening event. The stress response diminishes. You'll feel it after just a few breaths.

Once you feel yourself calming down, go through a mental checklist. Remember, you think more clearly once you have turned off the stress response since the higher blood flow to the cerebral cortical areas allows for more complex thought. So first take a few deep breaths. Then ask yourself whether this is really a life-threatening event. It's true that whatever is going on may not be according to how you would have written the script. It may be a major setback. But in the whole scheme of life, it usually isn't life-threatening or even that big a deal.

Next, ask yourself if you even have any control over what's happening. Much of what people stress about is out of their control. Other people may behave badly. Things may happen that you wish hadn't. But you can't control that. *All you can control is how you choose to respond.* There is real freedom in realizing that you can't control a lot of what happens in life but that's okay. As the famous Serenity Prayer reads, "God grant me the serenity to accept the things I cannot change; courage to change the things I can; and wisdom to know the difference." Accepting that life is not perfect can be very freeing. As a dear friend of mine is fond of saying, "It is what it is. It's not bad. It's not good. It just is."

Of course, sometimes something stressful happens and you *do* feel you can have some control over the outcome. Maybe it is a project you are working on, or maybe something went wrong and you don't know how to handle it. *Write about it.* Just the process of writing down how you feel about something is helpful. You don't need to keep your notes. The process of expressing your feelings in writing engages more of your brain than just thinking about it does. Keeping a journal can be a very empowering way for you to see the problem from a different perspective; it often helps you to solve the problem. And remember, when you are calm, you have more blood flow to the area of your brain that allows you to think. So take a few slow, deep breaths at the start.

Try progressive muscle relaxation (where you progressively tighten and then relax individual muscle groups) and **visual imagery** (where you imagine being in a calm, peaceful setting doing something you find peaceful and enjoyable), which are two great stress relievers. Stay away from unhealthy coping strategies for stress such as overeating, smoking, alcohol, and recreational drugs. These will not help you in the long run.

Life can be stressful, no doubt about it, but keep going back to what is really important to you and try to focus on that instead of on the little things that go wrong. Stress management is an inside job. Because you can think yourself into the stress response, you can just as easily think yourself out of it. And you can learn how to be in charge of your emotions and thoughts far more than you ever thought possible. It will take practice, of course. It is all about repeating thoughts and behaviors. The more you do something, either a physical activity or a way of thinking, the more your neurons will cement their connections to one another and construct new pathways in your brain. There is a saying in the neuroscience world, "Neurons that fire together, wire together." You can physically (and I mean that literally) reset your brain so that you feel calmer, have a much longer fuse, and, yes, feel happier.

This week, try to identify the stressors in your life. What physical symptoms do you experience when you are stressed? Does your stomach hurt? Does your neck tighten? Do you have trouble sleeping? Make a list of a few long-term and short-term strategies for stress reduction that you would be willing to try over the next several weeks. Perhaps you can exercise, listen to music, run around outside with your kids, work in the garden, take a bubble bath, write about your feelings in a journal, watch the Comedy Channel. What strategies are you willing to try?

HEADACHES

Headaches are a common response to stress. The three most common types of headaches seen in an outpatient primary care setting are **muscular tension headaches, migraines,** and **temporomandibular joint pain**. These headaches have different causes, but the underlying initiator is often stress.

Stress can cause **muscular tension headaches** because the stress reaction (or fight-or-flight response) naturally causes your spine to tighten. Nature designed things so you wouldn't have a floppy spine if you were running away from a lion. Your spine muscles are connected to the muscles and connective tissue of your scalp, so your scalp muscles tighten, too, in stress and this can generate a headache. This kind of headache is often diffuse and described as "tight" or "squeezing."

Migraine headaches work differently. They are caused by blood vessels in the brain that first constrict and then overdilate. Since this increase in pressure is within a fixed area of your skull, you feel pain. Migraines typically cause nausea and vomiting; light and sound are also particularly bothersome. These headaches are intense, often throbbing and debilitating, and they may be preceded by flashing lights, blind areas of vision, or numbness and weakness on one side of the body. Migraines can be precipitated by stress, and they can also be precipitated by beverages and foods such as red wine and processed foods containing certain preservatives such as nitrates. They are also commonly precipitated by hormonal changes before a woman's menstrual cycle or in the perimenopausal period, when hormones fluctuate rapidly.

Temporomandibular joint (TMJ) pain is caused by inflammation in the small joint of the jaw, called the temporomandibular joint. This small joint can become inflamed if a person clenches or grinds his or her teeth at night or if the mouth remains open for long periods of time, such as at the dentist's. It can also become painful due to overuse from constant chewing or talking. Stress can also cause tightening of the TMJ muscle, causing pain. The TMJ joint often refers the pain to the scalp area, causing a headache. The TMJ joint is also right beside the ear, so people often describe the pain as coming from inside the ear. Treatment for TMJ pain includes stress relaxation measures, a night guard if teeth grinding is suspected, jaw rest by avoiding food that needs a lot of chewing, and anti-inflammatories such as ibuprofen when necessary.

NUTRITION: GETTING ORGANIZED

Eating well is possible even if you have a busy, hectic life. You *can* eat healthfully, but it does take a little planning and strategizing. Let's focus on how to keep healthful food in your life, even when you are on a tight schedule. In Week 8, we will review what to do when you eat out at a restaurant, go to parties, or travel a lot.

Let's start by talking about how to bring healthy food into your life. Rule number one: Keep healthy food *in* the house—and junk food *out*. We talked about this in Week 1, but this is crucial if you want to stick with a healthful eating plan. It does take a little effort, but it doesn't have to require a lot. Here's what you have to do:

- **Create your personal stock grocery list** by referring to our example of a healthy stock grocery list below. Feel free to modify it. Write down the fruits and vegetables you love. Decide what whole grains will be your staples. Pick some healthful snacks. Having a stock grocery list doesn't confine you to just these foods. It simply makes it easier to buy groceries because you don't have to re-create the list every time you go.

- **Keep a copy of your stock grocery list in your wallet or purse** or on your PDA so that you always have it for quick reference before your grocery run.

- **Plan exactly *when* you will go grocery shopping.** Pick a day each week when you will do your major shopping. Or if you like to pick up fresh food every day, decide what time you'll go every day. Try to plan ahead to avoid last-minute runs to the store.

- **Eat a snack before you go** so you never shop on an empty stomach.

- **Stick to your list!** Avoid impulse buying.

STOCK GROCERY LIST

GRAINS

BREAD

- ☐ 100% whole wheat with 2 or more grams of fiber per slice
- ☐ Corn tortillas
- ☐ Tortillas, whole wheat
- ☐ Whole-wheat bagels
- ☐ Whole-wheat crackers
- ☐ Whole-wheat English muffins
- ☐ Whole-wheat pitas

CEREAL

- ☐ Flaxseed meal
- ☐ Granola, low fat
- ☐ Oatmeal
- ☐ Wheat germ
- ☐ Whole-grain cereal with 3 or more grams of fiber per serving

DRIED

- ☐ Brown rice
- ☐ Bulgur
- ☐ Couscous
- ☐ Quinoa
- ☐ Whole-wheat pasta

FROZEN

- ☐ Reduced-fat pancakes, French toast, or waffles

FRUITS

FRESH

- ☐ Apples
- ☐ Bananas
- ☐ Blackberries
- ☐ Blueberries
- ☐ Cherries
- ☐ Clementines
- ☐ Grapefruit
- ☐ Grapes
- ☐ Lemons
- ☐ Limes
- ☐ Melons
- ☐ Nectarines
- ☐ Oranges
- ☐ Peaches
- ☐ Plums
- ☐ Strawberries
- ☐ Watermelon

Shopping Tips

- *Check off the foods you would like to purchase.*
- *Use this list to create your own personal shopping list on a separate piece of paper.*
- *Plan your meals around fruits, vegetables, whole grains, and lean meats.*
- *Fill half your shopping cart with fresh produce.*

DRIED OR CANNED

- ☐ Applesauce, unsweetened
- ☐ Dried fruit
- ☐ Orange juice with calcium
- ☐ 100% fruit juice

FROZEN

- ☐ Frozen fruits

VEGETABLES

FRESH

- ☐ Asparagus
- ☐ Avocados
- ☐ Beets
- ☐ Broccoli
- ☐ Brussels sprouts
- ☐ Cabbage
- ☐ Carrots
- ☐ Cauliflower
- ☐ Celery
- ☐ Corn
- ☐ Cucumber
- ☐ Eggplant
- ☐ Lettuce
- ☐ Mushrooms
- ☐ Onions
- ☐ Potatoes
- ☐ Spinach
- ☐ Squash
- ☐ Tomatoes
- ☐ Zucchini

CANNED

- ☐ Canned vegetables

FROZEN

- ☐ Broccoli
- ☐ Brussels sprouts
- ☐ Corn
- ☐ Edamame
- ☐ Peas and carrots
- ☐ Spinach
- ☐ Vegetable medley

DAIRY PRODUCTS

FRESH

- ☐ Cheese, low fat
- ☐ Cheese shreds, low fat
- ☐ Cottage cheese, low fat
- ☐ Milk, skim or 1%
- ☐ Parmesan cheese
- ☐ Soy milk, nonfat, low fat, or light
- ☐ Yogurt, nonfat
- ☐ Yogurt smoothies, light

FROZEN

- ☐ Frozen yogurt, low fat

MEAT OR MEAT SUBSTITUTES

FRESH

- ☐ Canadian bacon
- ☐ Chicken breast
- ☐ Egg substitutes
- ☐ Eggs
- ☐ Fish
- ☐ Lean beef or other meats
- ☐ Tempeh
- ☐ Tofu
- ☐ Turkey bacon
- ☐ Turkey breast

DRIED OR CANNED

- ☐ Almonds
- ☐ Black beans
- ☐ Garbanzo beans
- ☐ Kidney beans
- ☐ Lentils
- ☐ Nuts, mixed
- ☐ Peanut butter
- ☐ Peanuts
- ☐ Pinto beans
- ☐ Tuna fish in water
- ☐ Walnuts

FROZEN

- ☐ Vegetable burgers

FATS

- ☐ Butter
- ☐ Canola oil
- ☐ Cream cheese, light
- ☐ Margarine spread, low fat and trans fat free
- ☐ Mayonnaise, reduced fat
- ☐ Olive oil
- ☐ Olives
- ☐ Salad dressing
- ☐ Sour cream, nonfat

SWEETS AND TREATS

- ☐ Cocoa powder, sugar free
- ☐ Cookies, low fat
- ☐ Popsicles, fat free, no sugar added
- ☐ Pudding, nonfat

COMBINATION FOODS

- ☐ Chili, canned
- ☐ Healthy frozen entrées
- ☐ Soup, low fat

MISCELLANEOUS

CONDIMENTS AND MARINADES

(compare brands to find those low in salt or salt free)

- ☐ Chicken broth
- ☐ Jelly, sugar free
- ☐ Ketchup
- ☐ Mustard
- ☐ Nonstick cooking spray
- ☐ Salsas
- ☐ Soy sauce, light
- ☐ Spices
- ☐ Tomato paste
- ☐ Tomato sauce

Let's go through a mock grocery run. First, eat a little snack before you go. Get your grocery list. Now let's walk through all the different food aisles.

FRUITS

Fresh fruits in season offer the best value and taste. Fresh is better than canned, especially if canned means that the fruit is packed in syrup. Frozen fruits are almost as good as fresh, so stock up on them and keep them in the freezer. Frozen fruit is great for making smoothies or frozen fruit snacks. Include dried fruit, too, if you like it. Just watch the serving sizes when you eat dried fruit, because the calories are very concentrated. If you buy fruit juice, make sure it is 100% fruit juice and not flavored sugar syrup.

VEGETABLES

Fresh vegetables in season offer the best value and taste. Frozen vegetables run a close second to fresh vegetables in nutritional value. Keep them in the freezer so you can quickly throw them into stir-fries, stews, or casseroles. Canned vegetables are generally loaded with salt, so they are not a good choice. Aim for a variety of colors to get a variety of nutrients.

GRAINS

Choose whole-grain products. If they aren't whole grain, you don't want them. Look for whole-grain cereals and breads with 2 or more grams of fiber per serving. Choose whole-grain crackers with low fat and sodium content.

PROTEIN

Your best protein sources are plant products (such as legumes, lentils, nuts, and seeds) and fish. If you like animal meat, eat beef sparingly, as it is the highest in saturated fat of all meats. The healthiest grades of meat are select and choice, and the healthiest cuts are round, loin, and flank. Ground beef should be over 90% lean. Ground turkey is better than ground beef, but only if the turkey has been ground without the skin (otherwise it is no better). Ground turkey made from white meat is also lower in fat than ground turkey with dark meat. If you choose canned tuna, it should be packed in water, not oil. Also, light tuna contains less mercury than the larger, tuna-like albacore. Soy hot dogs or any soy or tofu meat substitutes are good options because plant-based protein contains healthy, unsaturated fat.

DAIRY PRODUCTS

Here you need to concentrate on taking the fat out. Dairy products all contain a lot of saturated fat, and our digestive system doesn't handle this type of fat well, so you should be choosing nonfat yogurt and nonfat milk. Buy nonfat or low-fat cottage cheese. Go easy on regular cheese. If you want to have a little cheese on something to bring out the flavor, buy a cheese that has a strong flavor so you need to use only a little. Use nonfat or low-fat cheese whenever possible.

FATS AND OILS

Choose olive oil or canola oil to get the best nutrition. Use a cooking spray when you can to save calories. Choose lower-fat dressings and ones that contain unsaturated fats, such as a balsamic/olive oil vinaigrette rather than a more saturated fat option such as blue cheese dressing. Skip butter (which contains saturated fat) and margarine (which usually contains unhealthy trans fats). A few butter substitutes do not contain saturated or trans fats, but you'll have to read the label to be sure. You can also substitute olive oil for butter in many dishes.

How to Read a Food Label

Once you master the basic ground rules for healthy grocery shopping, start to focus on reading food labels. When you buy something that is packaged, you should look at the list of ingredients. By law, the ingredients must be listed on the label in order of weight. *The first ingredient is highest in weight.* The rest of the ingredients follow in descending order of weight. Reading labels is a way to make sure you aren't being slipped trans fat or a lot of extra sugar.

After you have looked at the list of ingredients, read what is meant by a

HOW TO READ A FOOD LABEL

The Nutrition Facts Label can help you make informed food choices for your healthy diet. Once you have learned how to use the label, you can very quickly decide if the food is a good choice. Follow the explanations below to understand each section of the label. All labels follow this format, with information about the specific product given in sections 1 to 4, and the same footnote (5), included on all labels.

Nutrition Facts

Serving Size 16 tiny crackers (130 g)
Servings Per Container about 9

Amount Per Serving

Calories 150   **Calories from Fat** 50

	% Daily Value*
Total Fat 6 g	9%
Saturated Fat 1 g	5%
Trans Fat 0 g	0%
Cholesterol 0 mg	0%
Sodium 260 mg	11%
Total Carbohydrate 21 g	7%
Dietary Fiber 1 g	4%
Sugars 4 g	
Protein 2 g	

Vitamin A 0%	Vitamin C 0%
Calcium 2%	Iron 6%

* Percent Daily Values are based on a 2,000 calorie diet. Your daily values may be higher or lower depending on your calorie needs.

	Calories	2,000	2,500
Total Fat	Less than	65 g	80 g
Sat Fat	Less than	20 g	25 g
Cholesterol	Less than	300 mg	300 mg
Sodium	Less than	2,400 mg	2,400 mg
Total Carbohydrate		300 g	375 g
Fiber		25 g	30 g

1 Start here.

2 Check calories.

3 Limit these nutrients.
Quick guide to % Daily Values:
▶ 5% or less is low
▶ 20% or more is high

4 Get enough of these nutrients.

5 Footnote.

1 Start here.

The first place to begin is with the serving size and the number of servings in the package. Serving sizes are standardized so you can easily compare similar foods. If you eat the equivalent of two servings, you must double the calories and nutrients.

2 Check calories.

This is the amount of calories per serving, using the correct serving size. When one serving of a food item has more than 400 calories per serving, it is high in calories. By looking at the calories and nutrients listed on the label, you can determine whether the food is worth eating.

Calories from fat: These are calories solely from fat. Focus on getting fat in your diet from monounsaturated and polyunsaturated fats. Skip food products that contain trans and saturated fats.

3 Limit these nutrients.

These are nutrients most people eat in adequate amounts or even too much of. Eating too much fat, saturated fat, trans fat, cholesterol, or sodium may increase your risk of certain chronic diseases, such as heart disease, some cancers, and high blood pressure.

Sugars refer to both natural and added sugars. Read the ingredients list to find added sugars, which may be listed as sugar, sucrose, glucose, high-fructose corn syrup, corn syrup, maple syrup, honey, and fructose. If sugar is among the first few ingredients, the food is high in added sugar. Since added sugar contributes empty calories, look for foods and beverages low in added sugars.

4 Get enough of these nutrients.

Most people have to work hard to get enough fiber, vitamin A, vitamin C, calcium, and iron in their diet. Eating the right amounts of these nutrients can help to prevent some diseases and conditions. Foods with 5 grams of fiber or more are considered "high-fiber" foods. Vitamins and minerals are shown as percentages. The goal is to consume 100% of each of these nutrients daily to prevent nutrition-related diseases.

5 Footnote.

The statement "*Percent Daily Values are based on a 2,000 calorie diet" must appear on all food labels. If the package is small, the rest of this section may not appear. The full footnote is always the same, because it shows recommended dietary advice, not information about the food in the package. Daily Values are recommended levels of intakes. They are shown for a 2,000-calorie and a 2,500-calorie diet.

serving size and how many servings are in each container so you are not misled by the quantity of food it is referring to.

Next, look at the total calories and check how many calories are coming from fat. In general, a quarter or a third of our calories should come from fat, so if it is more than this, the food is high in fat. More important, you should see what *kind* of fat it contains; unsaturated fats are good, while saturated and trans fats are bad. A little saturated fat is okay, but you should really try to avoid trans fats entirely. Food companies list trans fat as zero if they can. They are legally allowed to list trans fats as zero on the label if there is less than .5 gram of trans fat in each serving. What you want is no trans fat at all. When you read the list of ingredients, check to see if it includes partially hydrogenated vegetable oil. This is trans fat.

Also, look at the amount of fiber in each serving. You are trying to get 25 to 35 grams of fiber per day, so anything with 3 or more grams of fiber per serving is good. That's the amount you would get in a typical serving of a fruit or vegetable.

The sugars on the food label refer to both natural and added sugars. The number of sugar grams listed needs to be taken within its context. A pure fruit contains sugar, but it is natural and healthy if eaten whole. Fruit also contains fiber, which will absorb the natural sugar slowly. Fruit juice is without fiber, however, and has the same natural sugar content but no fiber to help in absorbing the sugar slowly. Fruit juice is therefore something to consume in moderation. If you read the ingredients list and sugar has been added to the food, that's not good. Sugar goes by the names sugar, sucrose, glucose, high-fructose corn syrup, corn syrup, maple syrup, honey, and fructose.

Reading labels can be quick. You don't need to look at every piece of data on the label; just focus on the serving size and calories, the type of fat, and whether the food contains fiber, or just go straight to the ingredients list on the label and see which ingredients are highest in abundance. Remember, ingredients are listed in order of weight, from highest to lowest. It is important to use food labels not only to limit the nutrients you want to cut back on but also to focus on the nutrients you want to increase in your diet, such as fiber and calcium. Food labels can be a big help when you pick up an unfamiliar food and want to see if it is a healthful choice.

Quick tips for reading a Nutrition Facts label:

- Begin by reading how many servings the package contains and the calories per serving.

- Avoid foods with trans fat and saturated fat.

- Check the cholesterol content. Less than 20 milligrams per serving is considered low.

- Limit sodium. Less than 140 milligrams per serving is considered low.

- Pick foods with fiber, ideally more than 5 grams per serving. Remember, any amount of fiber is beneficial.

Making Sense of Food Label Terms

Fat-free: Product has less than 1/2 gram of fat per serving.

99% fat-free: Every 100 grams of food will have 1 gram or less of fat.

Low-fat: Product has 3 grams or less of fat per serving.

Reduced-fat: Fat has been reduced by at least 25% when compared with a similar food product.

Light: Product has 33% fewer calories or 50% less fat per serving than a comparable product.

Lean: Used for meat and poultry only. Product has less than 10 grams of fat, less than 4 grams of saturated fat, and less than 95 milligrams of cholesterol per serving.

Low-calorie: Product has 40 calories or less per serving.

Saturated fat free: Product has less than 0.5 gram of saturated fat per serving.

Trans fat free: Product has less than 0.5 gram of trans fat per serving.

Low in saturated fat: Product has 1 gram or less of saturated fat per serving.

Cholesterol-free: Product has less than 2 milligrams of cholesterol per serving.

Low-cholesterol: Product has less than 20 milligrams of cholesterol and 2 grams of saturated fat per serving.

Sodium-free: Product has less than 5 milligrams of sodium per serving.

Very low sodium: Product has 35 milligrams or less of sodium per serving.

Low-sodium: Product has 140 milligrams or less of sodium per serving.

Good source of: Used for fiber, protein, vitamins, or minerals. Product has at least 10% of the Daily Value of a particular nutrient.

High in (Excellent source of): Used for fiber, protein, vitamins, or minerals. Product has at least 20% of the Daily Value of a particular nutrient.

STAYING HEALTHY ON THE ROAD

When you travel a lot, whether for business or vacation, it can seem harder to stay healthy because it's harder to stay on a routine. But you *can* do it; you just have to pay a little more attention to your food choices, food portions, and physical activity level. Here are several tips people find helpful for staying on track.

- Deli sandwiches can be a good option when you are traveling. Choose whole-wheat bread; substitute mustard for mayonnaise; choose lean-meat fillings such as lean roast beef or turkey; save extra calories by skipping the cheese; add lettuce, tomato, or other veggie toppings to help meet your daily vegetable needs.

- For long car or train rides or plane flights that don't include meals, pack some healthy snacks such as fresh or dried fruit, whole-wheat crackers, or energy bars. Take a bag of fresh, crunchy bite-size vegetables along. These are all high in fiber and may also help if you suffer from constipation when traveling. Nuts in single serving packets are another good option to keep hunger under control. Bring bottled water and keep it cold in an ice chest if you're driving.

- When you are flying, be sure to drink plenty of water, as the air in the plane is dehydrating. Avoid alcohol and caffeine, which act as diuretics and can contribute to dehydration.

- When you are traveling across several time zones, try to adapt to the new time as quickly as possible, including mealtimes. This will help you stick with your healthful eating routines.

- Eating out all the time can be tricky, but make the most healthful choices you can and focus on portion control.

- If you'll be visiting an exotic place, take time to research the health precautions for that area. Know whether the food and water are safe and whether certain vaccines are recommended. The Centers for Disease Control and Prevention (CDC) website is great for this.

- Finally, don't forget to exercise. If you are sightseeing, try to walk to see the sights whenever possible. If you are traveling on business, use the hotel gym or pack a lightweight resistance band or jump rope. You can even buy weights that require you to add water to provide the weight. Then you just drain out the water when it's time to pack up and travel again.

- One Program participant joined the YMCA and made it a challenge to go to the local "Y" wherever he went on a business trip. He treated it like an adventure.

- Pack your running shoes on top of your clothes so they will be in plain view when you open your suitcase.

You *can* stay healthy when you are traveling. You may have to be a little more creative about it, but chances are, if you're feeling healthy, you'll be more likely to have a great trip.

FITNESS: IMPROVING YOUR CARDIORESPIRATORY FITNESS

Now let's take a look at how you can achieve greater cardiorespiratory fitness. First let me define what I mean by this. Optimal cardiorespiratory fitness means your body has learned to do three things:

- Your lungs have learned to be efficient in extracting oxygen from the air and eliminating carbon dioxide waste from your body.

- Your heart has learned to be efficient in pumping oxygen-filled blood quickly throughout the body.

- Your muscles have learned to extract large amounts of oxygen from the blood so that large amounts of adenosine triphosphate can be created as an energy source.

Cardiorespiratory fitness is measured by assessing VO_2 max, which is a measure of how much oxygen your body absorbs and utilizes during peak exercise. The higher the VO_2 max, the better your fitness.

You don't need to have a complicated plan for increasing your cardiorespiratory or aerobic fitness. You just need to be consistent with your exercise frequency, and you need to ramp up the intensity of aerobic activity at least three times a week. As we've talked about before, you should have your half-hour brisk walk (or an equivalent moderate-intensity aerobic exercise) every day as your foundation for fitness, but on three days per week increase the intensity and length of the walk (or workout) by an additional 20 to 30 minutes. During those longer sessions, vary the intensity. Speed up for a few minutes, then slow down for a few minutes. Repeat. Don't push yourself so much that you don't enjoy it, but do push yourself some to teach your body to be a little more prepared the next time you exercise. Your body will adapt quickly. It will say, "Hey, that was hard! I need to make a few changes here so I can handle this work better next time." And it will. Don't do high-intensity training more than five days a week, as this is associated with an increase in musculoskeletal injuries. Moderate-intensity exercise such as brisk walking can be done safely every day.

What does "pushing yourself" actually mean when it comes to heart rate? How high should you try to push your heart rate when you are working to increase your aerobic fitness? The general guideline to follow is that you should try to maintain your heart rate at 60 to 80 percent of your maximum heart rate for 20 to 60 minutes three to five times per week. That means if you have a base walk of 30 minutes a day, you should add 20 to 30 minutes a few times a week, during which you achieve higher heart rates of 60 to 80 percent of your maximum. Your base walk of three to four miles per hour typically gives you only a 50 percent maximum heart rate range.

As you know, to find your maximum heart rate, you can use the formula *maximum heart rate equals 220 minus your age.* You can also estimate your target heart rate by simply walking or running until you feel you are at an 8 on a 1-to-10 scale with 0 being at rest and 10 being how you feel when you have pushed yourself as hard as you possibly can. When you reach 8 on this perceived exertion scale, check your pulse. This heart rate is your 80 percent maximum heart rate. You will find that as you become more and more aerobically fit, your target heart rate will not change, but you will need to exert yourself more to get to that heart rate. Also, the speed with which your pulse drops down to normal after exercise increases the more fit you become.

For example, if you are 60 years old, your maximum heart rate is 160 (220 minus your age equals your maximum heart rate), so three times a week, you want to get your heart rate to 96 to 128 and hold it there for at least 20 minutes. Or if you are 20 years old, which means your maximum heart rate is 200, you should be getting your heart rate up to about 120 to 160 for at least 20 minutes three times a week. The 20 minutes is in addition to your 30-minute baseline exercise of brisk walking (or whatever base aerobic activity you prefer).

Now here's an extra bonus for those of you trying to lose weight. The higher your VO_2 max or aerobic fitness, the more calories you will burn with each workout. So not only will you burn calories while you work to achieve greater aerobic fitness, *you will burn even more calories as you become more fit!*

This week, keep on doing your 30-minute base walk (or whichever moderate aerobic activity you like best), but now add on 20 to 30 minutes three times a week at an increased intensity to improve your overall fitness and reap even more health benefits.

LEARN IT!

- Stress is a physiologic response to an event; it is not the event itself.

- Chronic stress increases your risk of heart disease, stroke, high blood pressure, obesity, and depression, so managing stress is crucial to your health.

- Stress in short bursts is not unhealthy and can even help your brain, but you need to know how to turn stress off so it does not become chronic.

- Your thoughts alone can turn the stress response on; your thoughts alone can also turn the stress response off.

- Exercise is one of the most proven, effective ways to manage stress.

- To increase aerobic (cardiorespiratory) fitness, do higher-intensity workouts that get you up to 60 to 80 percent of your maximum heart rate for at least 20 to 30 minutes three times a week. This should be in addition to your base activity of 30 minutes a day.

PERSONALIZE IT!

This week, work on your Emotional Brain.

The rational and emotional centers of your brain are tightly interconnected. This means your emotions can influence your behavior, and that can be either good or bad. You can learn how to modify your mood and stress levels in positive ways through various well-defined behaviors that improve your ability to stay healthy and happy.

Here are some examples of how people in The Program have personalized this brain principle and put it into action.

- Tom T., a 54-year-old business executive, found deep breathing exercises to be quite helpful when he was feeling stressed. During a particularly stressful meeting at work he would quietly take some slow, deep breaths to calm himself. He became known at his company as the "Rock of Gibraltar" because he was so good at remaining levelheaded and calm during the tense financial times the company was going through.

- Greta P., a 25-year-old high-tech project manager, had trouble unwinding when she came home from work each night. She continued to work on her computer, checking e-mails and working on projects until late every night. Greta decided to draw a clear line between work and home, so, except on rare occasions, when she came home each night, she put on music, ate dinner, took a bath, and read the newspaper by the fire. She did not let herself turn on the computer to do work-related tasks when she was at home, and she went to bed by 10 P.M. She also let herself unwind by watching a television sitcom that she had previously felt was a frivolous waste of time but secretly enjoyed. With these strategies, Greta learned that she had far more control over her negative emotions than she had previously thought.

- Alex A., a 43-year-old policeman, found that when he came home from work stressed and irritable every day, he used food and alcohol to unwind. He was struggling with a recent 30-pound weight gain, and he was becoming concerned about his alcohol intake. Alex learned that if he went for a run at the end of each day, he could relax without resorting to food and alcohol. Alex eventually lost 20 pounds, but his biggest success was that he felt a lot happier and closer to his family. Alex learned to manage his negative emotions rather than allow his negative emotions to manage him.

- Christopher A., a 34-year-old marketing consultant, struggled with feeling anxious about even small things in his life. He taught himself how to stop frequently throughout the day to do a few minutes of slow, deep breathing while he practiced thinking about things for which he felt deep appreciation. After some practice, he was able to quickly switch from feelings of anxiety to feelings of joy and gratitude, and this made him much happier and less anxious. Just knowing that he was more in control of his stress response helped him keep his anxiety in check.

LIVE IT!

- Review last week's goals and create this week's short-term goals.

- Pay attention to the things that create stress for you and choose a few short-term and long-term strategies to try.

- Design your own personal Stock Grocery List.

- Practice reading food labels.

- Add three 20-minute sessions of higher-intensity exercise each week to your baseline 30 minutes a day of moderate activity.

MAXIMIZING ENERGY

If there is no struggle, there is no progress.

—FREDERICK DOUGLASS

ARE YOU EXHAUSTED as you go through your day? Do you require lots of caffeine to keep you going? Persistent fatigue is one of the most common reasons people see a physician. There are many causes of fatigue; however, it is pretty common for a thorough medical evaluation to reveal nothing. This can be frustrating for patients because they feel as if nothing can be done to help them get their old energy level back.

Let's take a look at the causes of fatigue so you can begin to take the necessary steps for regaining your energy.

If you see your doctor about fatigue, he or she will focus on trying to find any underlying disease that might be the culprit. Thyroid disease, diabetes, adrenal insufficiency, anemia, allergies, fibromyalgia, multiple sclerosis, infection— these are all conditions associated with fatigue. A careful history, physical exam, and laboratory work should uncover these medical conditions if one exists. If a cause is found, of course, then treatment for the fatigue would begin by treating this medical condition. But what if everything appears normal? What might be other causes of fatigue?

Are you simply trying to do too much? The first obvious step is to look at the workload you face on a typical day. Are there so many tugs on your energy (work, children, aging parents, for example) that you have no time to nurture yourself, no time to "refuel"? Everyone needs some downtime to replenish energy stores, but we live in a world that moves faster than ever before and where expectations can feel so high that many of us feel that we need to run just to keep up. Sometimes all it takes to restore our energy is to learn how to say no or how to delegate.

Are you eating right? Take a close look at your eating habits, and you may discover some clues about why you feel so sluggish. Food is broken down into sugar units (or partially broken down sugar units) that combine with oxygen to make the body's energy currency, which is called adenosine triphosphate (ATP). ATP is the energy block that runs all the processes of your body, including your brain's ability to think. Your body does not store large amounts of ATP in your cells. You need to constantly make ATP from either sugar you have stored (glycogen in your liver and muscles) or from the food you eat. You can use fat from your fat stores to make ATP, but the body takes longer to do it this way and the stores are therefore not used as efficiently.

The best way to eat to provide for maximum energy is to have four to five small, frequent meals per day so that the body and brain will have constant access to glucose (sugar). The trick here is to take in small amounts so your body doesn't have more than it needs; otherwise it will convert the excess calories into fat. The other trick is to make sure you consume foods with high-fiber, complex carbohydrates that contain some protein and perhaps a little unsaturated fat but are not high in simple carbohydrates (sugar) or refined carbohydrates (for instance, white bread and rice), because that will give you a rapid blood sugar spike that will leave you hungry and exhausted after about two hours.

It's also important to have a diet that is varied and balanced that will give you all the vitamins and minerals you need. It is best if you can get all your nutrients from the food you eat, but if you have any doubt about that, take a multivitamin. If you are a woman who is menstruating, you may want to take a multivitamin with iron so you do not run the chance of developing iron-deficiency anemia because of the iron loss from your periods each month. Liver, eggs, rice, and beans are also sources of iron. Make sure you drink enough water, too. Hydration is important. Subtle feelings of fatigue sometimes stem from mild to moderate dehydration.

What about caffeine? In small doses, caffeine increases your concentration and reaction time and your brain cells actually fire more rapidly. If you do drink caffeine, though, it's important not to overdo it, or your body will go into overdrive, leading to palpitations, tremulousness, nervousness, and diarrhea. Most people should limit caffeine consumption to the hours before noon because the half-life of caffeine can be as long as 7 to 12 hours so there may be too much caffeine in your system for you to sleep well if you drink it too late in the day.

Are you getting enough sleep? What time do you go to bed at night? What time do you get up? Do you fall asleep quickly? Do you wake up frequently throughout the night? Do you smoke? Nicotine is stimulating. Do you drink alcohol at night? Alcohol disrupts sleep. Do you drink caffeine in the afternoon or evening? There are many things you can do to treat insomnia, so if this is a problem for you, it is important to identify it. If you fall asleep during the day, particularly if you are overweight or snore, you should get checked for sleep apnea. Sleep apnea is a condition in which the upper airway periodically closes off during sleep. People often don't know they have sleep apnea; they just know they feel exhausted all the time.

Are you depressed, stressed, or anxious? Many doctors feel that "emotional fatigue" may be the most energy-draining cause of fatigue there is. If you feel this is where the source of your fatigue may lie, it is important to have a well-delineated plan for treatment through stress reduction techniques, medication, counseling, or all three. Daily exercise can also be an enormous benefit in depression. I'll discuss mood in detail in chapter 8.

Sometimes people describe fatigue when they really mean lack of motivation. It isn't depression, but it is a type of apathy in which they do not feel passionate about anything anymore. Being excited about what you are doing is a huge energy booster, and sometimes the answer lies in brainstorming about things you used to be interested in but perhaps had to drop because your life got too busy. Dusting off old dreams and passions, finding new interests, challenges, and goals, can be the ticket to restoring energy.

Chronic inflammation can cause fatigue. Some of the newest research deals with inflammation, which appears to be responsible for the bulk of disease processes seen over time: heart disease, strokes, cancer, arthritis, dementia—even the aging process itself. It is also a reason for some people's fatigue. Chronic inflammation can occur when your well-meaning immune system gets a little carried away. Your immune system consists of patriotic fighting cells that attack foreign invaders. It is designed to protect you, but sometimes things go awry. For example, your immune system can attack whole organs in your body such as the pancreas (causing type 1 diabetes), your gut (causing ulcerative colitis or Crohn's disease), or your joints (causing rheumatoid arthritis). Even if your immune system is correctly fighting off foreign invaders, there can still be "friendly fire" that damages innocent bystander cells. A recent New Zealand study of 972 people showed higher inflammation markers in those with depression, too.

Most of the time, the outward effects of chronic inflammation are subtle and occur quietly beneath the surface of your body. Fatigue may be the only symptom.

Strategies for Increasing Energy

Your best strategy is to adopt a lifestyle that lets your immune system remain strong enough to fight true enemies but inactive when possible. Here's what we know today about how to help your immune system stay strong to maintain the right balance. **First, exercise.** This strengthens your immune cells and causes the production of a protein called sirtuin that decreases inflammation. It isn't easy at first—obviously, because you feel fatigued! But if you can push yourself to start, there are so many physiologic responses in the body that will increase your energy and stamina.

When you exercise, you train your body to be more efficient at utilizing the body's sugar sources to combine with oxygen to make ATP, so you will automatically have higher stamina levels. During exercise, the brain also secretes various neurotransmitters and chemicals that increase your mood and alertness level and make you less vulnerable to stress. Sleep is also improved by exercise because it enables you to get higher quantities of the deeper, more restorative sleep levels. **You should also strive to keep your weight normal** because fat cells secrete all kinds of chemicals that flame the inflammatory fire, accelerating aging and disease.

Next, choose healthful foods that keep inflammation in check. Fiber, for example, is very helpful for your immune system. Fiber sits in your gut and acts as a mesh to allow good bacteria to thrive and multiply, helping it keep the gut zone free from foreign invaders. Whole grains, fruits, and vegetables will supply you with fiber. Remember, animal products do not contain fiber. Fruits and vegetables are also an important part of your diet because they provide antioxidants that take the hit for the team by allowing their electrons to be snatched by free radicals so that the cell's electrons can be spared.

Unsaturated fats, specifically omega-3 fatty acids, a type of unsaturated fat, also fight inflammation. Omega-3 fatty acids are not as plentiful in the diet as omega-6 fatty acids (another type of unsaturated fat), so you usually have to go a bit out of your way to get them. Omega-3 fatty acids are in fatty fish (such as salmon), walnuts, and flaxseed. The ideal ratio of omega-3 to omega-6 is one to four, but I wouldn't get hung up on the numbers. If you feel you have risk factors for inflammation, it is not a bad idea to talk to your doctor about taking an omega-3 supplement. You can get omega-3 in fish oil capsules, in a dose of 1 to 3 grams a day. People do sometimes have trouble taking fish oil supplements because they can cause fishy breath. Here's a trick: store the fish oil supplements in the freezer and swallow the pills frozen. That will take care of the problem. Also, you should know that food choices that will work against you to promote bad-guy inflammatory cells are specifically saturated fat and particularly trans fat, as well as foods that are high in added sugar and processed, refined foods.

Alcohol (in moderation, of course) can be an anti-inflammatory, as can a daily aspirin. Ask your doctor before taking a daily aspirin, though, because it will increase your risk of bleeding a little. Aspirin has been shown to decrease arterial aging by 40 percent in those who take it daily.

Understand your normal biorhythms. All of us have an alertness and energy level that corresponds with our rising and falling body temperatures. The exact timing of your biorhythm is personal to you, but body temperature (and therefore alertness) is generally lowest at 4 A.M. It rises and peaks in the morning around 10 A.M. to 12 noon, then slumps somewhere between 2 and 4 P.M., at which time your body temperature rises and you get a second wind. Sometimes it helps to simply regulate energy-intensive tasks to peak energy times. And of course make sure you are getting enough sleep.

What about aging and energy loss? There are small but definite changes that happen in your body as you age. For example, did you know that once you hit 40, you cannot get into the deeper, more restorative stage four sleep? Also, after age 30, muscle mass starts to decline unless you use it. But these changes account for only a small loss of energy, and many (although not all) of these changes can be prevented or minimized with a healthy lifestyle. Exercise is an excellent way to lift energy levels.

To sum it all up, our energy levels are affected by many things in our lives, and we need to take a look at all of them. It is important to find time to relax and refuel, get adequate sleep and nutrition, fine-tune your stress management skills, rev yourself up with new goals and activities, and to work exercise into your routine. All these actions can make a difference in energy level and are worth trying if you suffer from fatigue that cannot otherwise be explained.

NUTRITION: WEIGHT LOSS STRATEGIES

Two thirds of Americans are considered overweight or obese. That's a huge number of people struggling with weight problems and the associated health problems. But Americans are working on it. At any given moment, one third of all Americans are on a diet.

Weight loss is a huge topic to try to cover in one week, but fortunately a lot of what you need to know to achieve and maintain a healthy weight is spread throughout The Program. Weight loss is certainly not just about food. It is also about how much you move, how well you sleep and handle stress, and how you think—it all matters. The following strategies for weight loss are based on those most frequently used by people who have not only lost substantial amounts of weight but have also kept it off.

Having a healthy body weight is very important to good health. Excess weight is second only to cigarette smoking for the amount of preventable disease and death it causes. The risk of developing heart disease, diabetes, cancer, strokes, high blood pressure, arthritis, sleep apnea, esophageal reflux, and gallstones increases dramatically for people who are overweight.

Before I list the top twenty strategies for weight loss, I want to point out one important fact that is spotted over and over again with successful weight losers: people who have lost substantial amounts of weight and kept it off have almost always made several unsuccessful attempts at weight loss before they finally succeeded. So if you have tried and failed before, don't be discouraged. Accept the fact that this in no way takes you out of the running. Success depends largely upon *resilience* and *persistence*.

As you review the strategies for weight loss that follows, realize that although some of these techniques have already been discussed and all of these recommendations may be familiar to you, they remain the most frequently used by those who have successfully lost weight and maintained this weight loss.

1   **Keep a food log.** Almost all successful weight losers do this. A food log helps you to be more conscious of what food you actually eat, and it helps you to spot patterns in your eating habits that are keys to long-term success. Food journaling is one of the most effective strategies of all for losing weight.

2   **Keep tempting food out of the house.** Keep healthful food available in both the home and workplace. When you are tired and hungry, it is just too difficult to get yourself to reach for healthful food if comforting but less healthful food is easily available.

3   **Practice portion control** at home and when eating out. Tips for portion control are covered in Week 10, but feel free to look ahead if this is an issue for you. Put your fork down after each bite. Enjoy the food you are eating. Take the time to taste it. Take note of whether you are hungry when you sit down to eat. How much does it really take to satisfy that hunger? Make it a habit to stop halfway through your meal for a break to talk for a while or reflect. It takes about twenty minutes for the chemicals in your body to trigger your brain's satiety center to turn off the drive to eat. At the very least, don't reach for seconds until you have waited twenty minutes.

4   **Read and understand food labels.** Choose food that is minimally processed, without added sugars or partially hydrogenated oils (trans fats). It's also best if the food is high in fiber. A food that is high in fiber is almost certainly minimally processed.

5   **Eat breakfast every morning, and don't skip meals.** People who eat breakfast tend to consume fewer calories on a daily basis than those who skip the morning meal. Those who are overweight tend to skip breakfast.

6 **Spread your calories out evenly throughout the day.** You should be eating at least four meals a day, and that good for everyone, whether you are trying to lose weight or not. Your brain needs a nice, even blood sugar level to keep your energy up and your mind alert. Studies clearly show that missing meals results in so much overeating at subsequent meals that people tend to actually gain weight. In other words, you aren't saving yourself calories when you skip meals, and your mental and physical performance suffers as well. Your best strategy for weight loss is to eat breakfast, lunch, a 4 P.M. snack, and dinner. If you don't eat a 4 P.M. snack, chances are that you will be so hungry at dinnertime that you will lose control and overeat. In fact, most people who are overweight eat little during the first half of the day and consume the majority of their calories in the evening.

7 **Eat plenty of fruits and vegetables each day.** Eating food that is bulky with fiber and water helps fill you up without dramatically increasing your calorie count. Fruit juice is not a great substitute for whole fruit; first, the fiber has been removed, and second, liquid calories are not as filling as calories from solid food, so you can easily go over your calorie threshold when you drink fruit juice.

8 **Eat a combination of complex carbohydrates and lean protein at each meal** so the rise in your blood sugar is slow and steady. If you eat refined or processed grains, your blood sugar rises and drops so fast that you become hungry in no time at all. But if you eat whole grains, they are absorbed much more slowly, so your feeling of satisfaction lasts longer. If you combine whole grains with protein, this satisfied feeling lasts even longer. Fat also gives you a very slow rise in blood sugar that lasts even longer, but remember, you probably don't have to go out of your way to find fat since it is already mixed into so many of the food groups.

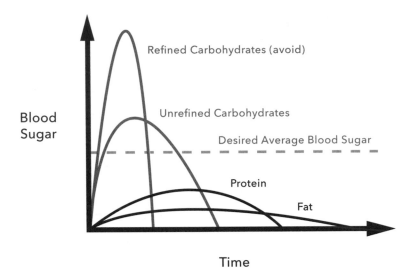

9 **Move your body more.** Unless you learn to move your body on an almost daily basis, the chance for permanent weight loss is poor. Regular exercise is the biggest predictor of long-term weight loss. The most popular physical activity for those who have successfully maintained weight loss is simply walking (45 to 60 minutes on average, most days of the week).

10 **Weigh yourself once a week.** If you want to weigh yourself every morning, go ahead, but daily weigh-ins can be somewhat discouraging because it takes a good week to see a pound or two of true weight loss. If you do weigh yourself daily, definitely avoid weighing yourself more than once a day. Nothing will happen that fast, and any variation you see within a day will just be a reflection of fluid shifts. In fact, weight varies by about three pounds throughout the day, the heaviest point usually being late in the afternoon.

11 **Anticipate high-risk food situations ahead of time and have a strategy to combat them.** Don't wait until you are in the thick of the fire (or the party) before planning an escape route. For example, if you know that Halloween night is going to be difficult because there will be candy around, chew gum while passing out candy to decrease your odds of

nibbling. Or consider buying Halloween candy that you don't like. Likewise, learn from your mistakes so you will have a strategy for the next time you are in the same situation. Losing weight is more about having a game plan than having willpower.

12 **Practice stress management techniques instead of relying on food for comfort.** Emotional eating is a major cause of weight gain. Have a list of activities you can do when you are feeling sad and tempted, so you are less likely to turn to food for comfort.

13 **Get enough sleep.** Studies show that people who shortchange their sleep needs are more likely to be overweight. Insufficient sleep leads to overproduction of certain hormones (cortisol, grehlin, and neuropeptide Y) that stimulate hunger and lead to overeating.

14 **Let go of the black-and-white way of thinking.** The all-or-nothing approach to weight loss is a recipe for failure. People who are trying to lose weight will have setbacks, but they need to get right back up and start again. You have to do this, too—forgive yourself and get on with it—if you want to succeed in the long run.

15 **Understand that weight loss is not the solution to all your problems.** There will always be things that bother you whether you lose weight or not, so don't be unrealistic. That will just lead to disappointment. Your life may be better, but not perfect, even if you lose all the weight you want.

16 **Keep your weight loss goal in perspective.** If the only way you define success is to have lost every inch of excess fat on your body, you are clearly setting yourself up for failure. For example, some people stop 5 or 10 pounds short of their ideal body weight because it is just too difficult to keep those final pounds off. That's okay. It doesn't negate the enormous health benefits gained from losing the other excess weight.

17 **Remember that you and only you are in the driver's seat.** Change has to come from you. You are the only one who can make it happen. No one can do it for you, and likewise, no one thing or person can sabotage your efforts to reach your goal. Only you can do that. Finally, you need to do what you are doing for yourself and not for anybody else.

18 **Don't feel you have to say good-bye to all desserts and treats forever.** Successful losers learn how to make peace with their most difficult temptations. Some people find it works for them to have just a nibble of their favorite treats when they want them, but others find they lose control too easily and do better restricting their favorite treats to certain special occasions that they specifically define ahead of time.

19 **Learn to speak to yourself in ways that help you to succeed rather than fail.** Speak to yourself positively, pat yourself on the back, and deal with setbacks in a positive, nonpunitive way. Believe that you can do it. Much of your ability to accomplish things in life lies in the power of believing you can do it. Look to people who have successfully maintained weight loss. Tell yourself, "If they can do it, so can I." And you can. Remember that whoever you think you are is often who you become. Use this to your advantage.

20 **Learn to do it your way.** Everyone is different, and there is no cookie-cutter approach to weight loss. Sure, on one level it is about calories in and calories out, but how each person decides to control the calories consumed differs. That's okay. Pick the weight loss strategies that resonate with you. You may even come up with some of your own that aren't discussed here. That's great. They just have to work for you.

Modifying Recipes

If you like to cook and experiment with recipes, you're lucky because you will be able to have a lot more control over what you are eating. You can make substitutions in recipes that make the foods more healthful without sacrificing flavor. Here are some substitution tricks:

- When a recipe calls for fat (butter, margarine, or oil), you can substitute applesauce in a one-to-one ratio. Or you can add a fat (preferably olive or canola oil) but cut the amount in half; you will save 100 calories for every tablespoon of fat you eliminate.

- For sour cream, use nonfat sour cream or nonfat yogurt (or a mixture of the two).

- For mayonnaise, use light or nonfat mayonnaise.

- If cream is called for, use low-fat or nonfat milk or evaporated skim milk. You may need to decrease the amount of milk slightly, depending on the recipe.

- If you are watching the number of eggs you're eating, you can substitute two egg whites for every one egg that is called for. Or you can cut down on the number of whole eggs you would otherwise use by alternating every whole egg with two egg whites.

- When you sauté, you can use a nonstick cooking spray. If you are stir-frying, try putting just a little oil in the pan and then adding other liquids such as water, broth, tomato juice, fruit juice, or wine for added moisture.

- If cheese is in the recipe, use low-fat or nonfat cheese or select a cheese with 5 or fewer grams of fat per ounce. If you want the flavor of the real thing but not all the extra fat and calories, use only half the amount of cheese called for.

- If ground beef is in the recipe, use lean ground turkey (it should contain approximately 3 grams of fat and 55 calories or less per ounce). If you choose lean ground beef, reduce the amount by half and increase other items such as vegetables, pasta, or rice to bulk up the meal.

- If a recipe calls for baking chocolate, use 3 tablespoons of cocoa and 1 tablespoon of water or oil for every ounce of chocolate in the original recipe.

- Finally, have fun when you're cooking and don't limit yourself to just these ideas. I bet you'll find lots of people happy to sample your work and let you know how you did!

Personal Gram Targets

Some people are curious about how to calculate the number of carbohydrate, protein, and food grams they are getting in their diet. If this is too technical for you, feel free to skip this section. It isn't hard to understand, though. First, look at how many servings are allotted in your Personal Nutrition Plan (see the chart on page 70). Each plan is based on percentages of the major nutrients: carbohydrates, protein, and fat. This information is broken down to determine the number of daily servings from the various food groups you should eat. The traditional ratio of these macronutrients in the average American diet is approximately 50 to 55 percent carbohydrates, 15 percent protein, and 30 to 35 percent fat. Here's an example of how to figure out the number of grams of each macronutrient in an 1,800-calorie diet with these ratios.

1,800 CALORIES

55% carbohydrates	**1 gram carbohydrate = 4 calories**
15% protein	**1 gram protein = 4 calories**
30% fat	**1 gram fat = 9 calories**

CARBOHYDRATES

55% of 1,800 calories = 990 calories

990 calories ÷ 4 calories/gram = 248 grams carbohydrates

PROTEIN

15% of 1,800 calories = 270 calories

270 calories ÷ 4 calories/gram = 68 grams protein

FAT

30% of 1,800 calories = 540 calories

540 calories ÷ 9 calories/gram = 60 grams fat

In this example, in an 1,800-calorie diet, the average person would consume 248 grams of carbohydrates, 68 grams of protein, and 60 grams of fat.

In The Program's Personal Nutrition Plan, the calorie breakdown is approximately 50 percent carbohydrates, 25 percent protein, and 25 percent fat. Figure out how many grams of each macronutrient you are getting in your plan. As you look at food labels in the future, you can compare the content in the food with what your daily gram target is. Remember, you do not have to be exact about this. It simply allows you to place the gram amounts you see on serving labels into a context that you can understand according to your own personal diet.

Do your own calculation of how many grams of carbohydrates, fat, and protein you are getting in your Personal Nutrition Plan:

MY PERSONAL NUTRITION PLAN

DAILY CALORIES: _____

NUTRIENT PERCENTAGES OF THE PERSONAL NUTRITION PLAN

Carbohydrates	50%
Protein	25%
Fat	25%

CARBOHYDRATES

_____ total daily calories x 50% (or .5) = _____ carbohydrate calories

_____ daily carbohydrate calories ÷ 4 calories/gram

= _____ grams carbohydrates

PROTEIN

_____ total daily calories x 25% (or .25) = _____ protein calories

_____ daily protein calories ÷ 4 calories/gram

= _____ grams protein

FAT

_____ total daily calories x 25% (or .25) = _____ fat calories

_____ daily fat calories ÷ 9 calories/gram

= _____ grams fat

UNDERSTANDING YOUR PERSONAL NUTRITION PLAN

The following chart will help you get some idea of the number of grams per serving of carbohydrates, protein, and fat for each food group. Remember, a "serving" is the "serving size equivalent," not necessarily the portion of food on your plate.

FOOD GROUPS	CARBOHYDRATES (GRAMS)	PROTEIN (GRAMS)	FAT (GRAMS)	CALORIES
Grains	15	3	0–1	80
Fruits	15	0	0	60
Vegetables	6	.5	0	25
Dairy products*	12	8	0–3* (low-fat)	90
Meat or Meat Substitutes	0	21	0–9	150
Fat	0	0	5	45

*Dairy products (low-fat or nonfat) contain 0–3 grams of fat per serving, but whole dairy products, such as whole milk, contain 8 grams of fat per 1-cup serving.

Your plan is based on a specific number of servings of each group, with a total that will equal your daily calorie goal. The system works easily when simple foods are eaten, but many foods are a combination of different food groups. For example, lasagna is considered a combination food. It is typically composed of dairy product, grain, vegetable, and meat and/or fat. You can approximate how much of each food is included and make a guess to count the servings from each food group.

For packaged foods, you can simply refer to the Nutrition Facts label to learn how many grams (and equivalent servings) of each nutrient the product contains. At first this may seem confusing, but you will quickly get accustomed to reading labels and using the information to help you make decisions about the nutrient values of the foods that you are considering.

FITNESS: WHY BE STRONG?

This week we're going to talk about muscles. Muscles are made up of individual long muscle fibers, which are themselves made up of individual long muscle cells. When you lift weights or do resistance exercises, you create small tears in the muscles. In response to these tears, the fibers repair and grow back thicker and stronger in order to withstand future similar stress. It is therefore important to allow muscles to rest in between workout sessions because the muscles need time to repair and strengthen themselves. Allow at least a day between muscle-building sessions for individual muscle groups to heal.

Muscles are mostly genetically programmed, but they are also influenced by hormones such as testosterone, which makes muscles grow. Because women do not have high testosterone levels, they do not "bulk up" the way men do when they lift weights. Other hormones influence muscle mass, too. For example, cortisol (produced by stress) can cause muscles to atrophy if it is present in high amounts for long periods of time. Muscles will also grow if they feel they are needed, and this is where resistance exercise plays a role.

Your body doesn't want to spend the resources and energy necessary for a muscle's upkeep unless it sees that there is a need. That's just your body being smart and efficient. Muscle mass peaks in your twenties, but sometime in your thirties, your muscles start to atrophy unless you use them consistently. In today's world, where there are garage door openers, electric lawn mowers, and pretty much everything you can think of to keep you from having to use a muscle, it does require extra effort to keep your muscles from atrophying, let alone to increase their strength and tone.

Anybody who maintains a strong core muscle mass throughout life stands a much better chance of thriving in later years. In fact, the biggest predictor of whether an elderly person will be able to remain at home independently or will have to be placed in assisted living is whether his or her core muscles are still strong enough to allow him or her to perform normal activities of daily living (getting out of a chair, dressing, bathing) without having a high risk of falling.

Your muscles are important for many other reasons. For example, your metabolism is partly genetically programmed, but the amount of muscle on your body determines the level of your metabolism. For the same amount of weight, your muscles burn forty times as many calories as fat. Wow! Your muscles are calorie-burning machines! If you are trying to lose weight, your best offensive plan is to reduce calories while doing both aerobic exercise and strength-building resistance exercise. The aerobic exercise will burn more calories at any one exercise session, but the resistance exercises will build more muscle so that your overall resting metabolism will increase. This means that even when you are sleeping at night you will burn more calories. Now, that's pretty hard to beat!

If you are trying to lose weight, realize that muscle is dense and heavy, so if you are on a weight loss program and doing resistance exercises, you may lose inches before you lose pounds. Just be persistent; eventually you will lose pounds as well. Remember, too, that when you are reducing caloric from your diet, don't overdo it—don't go too low. If you reduce your caloric intake too much, your body will make up for the calorie deficit by burning both muscle and fat instead of just fat. You will notice that people who are starving don't have much muscle definition even though they have almost no fat. That is because the calorie deficit has been so severe that muscles have been sacrificed along with the fat. So *don't try to lose more than one to two pounds per week.*

Even if you have a reasonable calorie deficit, your body has a tendency to try to preserve some fat just in case starvation is looming around the corner. So if you don't do some muscle-building resistance exercises, your body will sacrifice some of your precious muscle to make up for the calorie debt. By doing resistance exercises, you are telling your body, "I'm sorry, these muscles are being used. You're going to have to make up the calorie debt somewhere else." Just show your body that you are using your muscles, and your body will not sacrifice them. You are in charge!

LEARN IT!

- Fatigue can be caused by lifestyle behaviors that promote chronic inflammation.

- Exercise is an excellent way to increase your energy level.

- The most common reasons for weight gain are lack of sufficient exercise and large food portions.

- There are twenty proven strategies that work in long-term weight loss.

- Muscle mass largely determines one's metabolism.

- Strong core muscles play a key role in whether an elderly person is able to remain independent in the later years of life.

PERSONALIZE IT!

This week, work on your Believing Brain.

Your brain is greatly influenced by whether you believe you can do something. In fact, simply believing in your ability to perform a task is as important as having the actual skill to do it. Your brain promotes a lot of behavior that reflects who you *think* you are. Use this to your advantage. Break large goals into small achievable steps. As you succeed with them your confidence will start to grow. Also, always believe in your best self, because, chances are, this is who you will become.

Here are some examples of how people in The Program have personalized this brain principle and put it into action.

- Annie S., a 43-year-old nurse, grew up thinking of herself as "fat and lazy," and her weight of 280 pounds convinced her that this was true. When she finally decided she was tired of dealing with the consequences of her weight, she began to power walk. During her power walks, she practiced goal visualization. She imagined herself as a strong, slim, athletic woman who was finally taking charge. Every day, she power walked longer and faster, and every day, she visualized herself as this strong, slim, athletic woman. Over time, her weight began to drop—first 20 pounds, then 30, and eventually 120 pounds! The incredible thing to her was that she eventually became the person she had seen in her mind's eye during her power walks—the woman she had been visualizing.

- Tony H., a 49-year-old computer programmer, grew up with a very athletic younger brother, and he described himself as "the opposite of my brother." Tony did not like to exercise. However, he needed to work on stress management and sleep problems, so he knew exercise would be important. Begrudgingly, he began an exercise program. Since his knees bothered him, he decided to take up swimming. At first he swam slowly and deliberately. Over time, though, he became pretty good at it. People started to notice how fast he did his laps. They would jokingly leave the lane whenever he entered, saying "I'm getting out of the way so I don't get run over." This really increased Tony's confidence, and he swam more. He joined a master's swim program. Now Tony considers himself an athlete—and he acts like one. He has the confidence and the physique of an athlete, but, more importantly, he lives like one.

- Priscilla T., a 38-year-old mother of three, used to view herself as impatient and short-tempered. When she became a mother for the first time, she decided to change this. She wanted to be patient and calm. She decided to take one small, easy step: she would simply wait fifteen seconds before responding to issues to which she would normally snap. What Priscilla found was that her fifteen-second rule allowed her to see a calmer, more patient version of herself. Most times, it allowed her to see that the issue was not really worth losing her temper over. In time she became calm and balanced, and her kids can't remember a time when she was short-tempered. They describe her as "the most patient mom around."

LIVE IT!

- Review last week's goals and create this week's short-term goals.

- Identify things in your life that may be sapping your energy or promoting inflammation.

- If you need to lose weight, identify the number one factor you feel has contributed to this problem. Choose a few weight loss strategies that you are willing to try.

- Take some time this week to think about how you view yourself. Are your belief systems about who you are helping you or making it more difficult to accomplish your goals?

OUTSMARTING HEART DISEASE

How we spend our days is, of course,
how we spend our lives.

–ANNIE DILLARD

EVERYONE KNOWS HOW important it is to have a healthy heart. Heart disease is, in fact, the leading cause of death in the United States. Fortunately, the kinds of things that contribute to heart disease are mainly lifestyle-related and very preventable, so this is an area where you can make a big difference. Although there are several different causes of heart disease, most are due to a buildup of plaque in the blood vessels (arteries) that feed the heart. Whenever the blood flow feeding an area of the heart is interrupted, this area of the heart dies. This is what we call a "heart attack."

It works like this: You have arteries that feed all of the organs in your body. Whether your kidneys or liver or heart or brain, all organs need to have blood flow to stay alive and function effectively. All of our arteries have three layers: a thin inner layer, a muscular middle layer, and a fibrous outer layer.

The inner layer acts as the front line for keeping the arteries healthy. This layer secretes chemicals that allow the arteries to dilate and constrict as needed; it also secretes chemicals that work to keep everything in your blood moving easily along. Unfortunately, there is a bad guy in this story, and he occasionally slips past the inner lining of the arteries into the muscular middle layer. This bad guy is called low-density lipoprotein (LDL) cholesterol. LDL is a small form of cholesterol, so it is particularly able to invade the inner lining when the lining has been injured.

How Much Does Your Heart Weigh? *If you are a woman, about 8 ounces; if you are a man, about 10 ounces.*

But what injures the inner lining in the first place? There are the injuries that come with wear and tear in all of us as we age, but several things greatly increase the number of injuries to the inner lining: high blood pressure, smoking, high blood sugar, and oxidized LDL cholesterol. All of these have the power to do significant damage to our precious arteries.

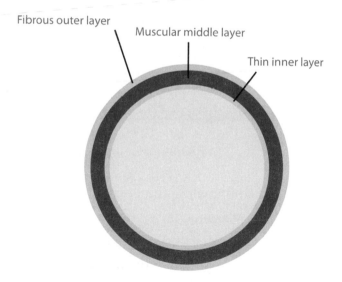

Fibrous outer layer
Muscular middle layer
Thin inner layer

What exactly is cholesterol? Cholesterol is an essential part of a cell membrane and is a necessary precursor to making numerous hormones. You get some cholesterol from the foods you eat, but most of your cholesterol is made in your liver. Saturated fats, and trans fats in particular, drive the production of LDL, which is referred to as "bad" cholesterol. It is bad because it promotes the buildup of plaque in your arteries. High-density lipoprotein (HDL) is referred to as "good" cholesterol because it pulls the bad LDL out of circulation, thereby helping to prevent the buildup of plaque.

The process of plaque buildup goes like this: First, the cells of the inner layer of the artery become injured, creating small nicks in the inner lining. These nicks may occur as a result of oxidized LDL, smoking, high blood sugar, or high blood pressure, as I've just mentioned. Once the nicks occur, it is much easier for LDL to slip past the inner lining of the artery into the middle layer. When LDL slips past the front line, a chemical alarm bell goes off,

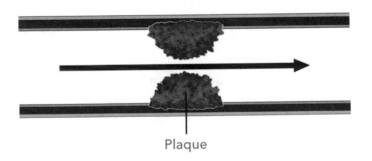

Plaque

announcing the presence of a foreign invader. The inflammatory system, acting as the police, becomes activated and rushes in to save the day.

Although the inflammatory system is designed to help, it ends up making a bit of a mess. It forms a soft, mushy plaque right over the area where the LDL has invaded. This does help to contain the problem, but the area becomes a hotbed of inflammation. Sticky platelets are a part of that inflammation.

Over time, the soft, unstable plaque will form a hard, fibrous cap. In the early stages, when the plaque is soft and unstable, there is a high possibility of plaque rupture. This is the cause of 75 percent of heart attacks. When a plaque ruptures, the area of rupture attracts even more inflammatory cells and sticky platelets. This can then trigger the formation of a clot that can suddenly and completely cut off the blood supply downstream.

Your Pulse *As a child, your resting pulse (heart beats per minute) is in the range of 90 to 120 beats per minute. As an adult, it slows down to an average of 72 beats per minute.*

You must realize that this process can be acute, as I just described, or it can go on for years. When the latter happens, new plaque is laid down on old plaque until the arteries allow only a trickle of blood to pass.

Sure, there are some things about this process you can't control. You have a higher risk of heart disease if you are male or have a family history of early heart disease. Your risk also increases as you age. With aging, over time, nicks inevitably occur in the arteries, but your body has a repair crew that can fix many of these insults. If you overwhelm the system, though, the repair crew cannot keep up. So how can you minimize the number of nicks in your arteries?

Circulation Fact
It takes about twenty seconds for blood to circulate throughout the entire vascular system.

- **First, do not smoke!** If you do only one thing for your health, make it smoking cessation. Cigarette smoke is extremely irritating to the inner lining of the arteries and therefore dramatically accelerates the process of plaque buildup. When you stop smoking, you significantly reduce your risk of heart disease. By the end of the first year your risk is reduced by half, and after fifteen years your risk is equal to that of someone who has never smoked. If you currently smoke, now is the time to think long and hard about whether you feel ready to stop. List

Cigarette Smoke

- *4,000-plus chemical compounds are found in cigarette smoke.*
- *200 of these are known to be poisons.*
- *60 have been identified as carcinogens.*

the advantages and disadvantages of smoking, and decide how you would score your motivation on a scale of 1 to 10. Consider setting a date to stop. For more information on prescription or nonprescription medication that can reduce cravings and withdrawal symptoms, as well as a list of the top twenty strategies to kick the habit, go now to Week 9, where this is discussed in more detail. You can also talk to your doctor. And you can get information and help by calling 1-877-937-7848, a free smoking cessation hotline provided by the American Cancer Society.

- **Keep your blood pressure less than 130/80—the lower the better.** Several recent studies show the risk of developing heart disease begins to climb when your blood pressure is above 115/75, so it's best to aim low. The top number in the reading is called the *systolic* pressure and measures the pressure inside your arteries at its maximum, when your heart initially pumps the blood with each heartbeat. The second number is the *diastolic* pressure, the pressure in your arteries when the heart is relaxed. Both are important. To lower your blood pressure, work to lose excess weight, exercise, minimize your salt intake, and avoid excess alcohol consumption. A diet high in fruits, vegetables, and whole grains also lowers blood pressure. This type of diet is called the Dietary Approaches to Stop Hypertension (DASH) diet. Take medication if needed. Don't neglect sleep, and avoid stress. Lack of sleep raises blood pressure, and so does stress. If you have high or borderline high blood pressure, buy a digital blood pressure cuff from a local pharmacy and get into the habit of checking your blood pressure regularly. Keep a log of your blood pressure.

- **Keep your blood sugar level normal.** A diabetic's risk of developing heart disease is proportional to his or her average blood sugar level. The goal for everyone's blood sugar level is less than 100 mg/dl (measured first thing in the morning after a twelve-hour fast). Excess blood sugar irritates the inner lining of the arteries by attaching to proteins on the inner wall. This irritation causes nicks in the lining and starts the process of plaque formation. You will learn more about how to control blood sugar with lifestyle changes in Week 6.

- **Keep your LDL cholesterol level less than 130 mg/dl—preferably less than 100 mg/dl,** especially if you have diabetes. If you have known heart disease, where your arteries are already filled with cholesterol plaques, you need to keep the LDL level at less than 70 mg/dl. You can do this through a reduction of body fat, regular exercise, and diet. Your diet should be low in saturated fat, trans fat, and cholesterol. It should be high in fiber and include unsaturated fats. Saturated fat comes from animal products and dairy products, so minimize your consumption of beef and pork and remove the skin from chicken and turkey. Fish are healthful because even the fattiest fish have mainly unsaturated healthy fats. Remember to consume low-fat dairy products as much as possible, and try to minimize your consumption of cheese and butter, which are often found in baked goods. Also, read labels so you can avoid foods high in "partially hydrogenated vegetable oil," a code phrase for trans fats. Those of you who need to lose some weight will be happy to know that the bad LDL cholesterol level usually drops dramatically with weight loss. You may need to take medication if you were simply born with a liver that is too efficient an LDL production factory. Recent research suggests that it may be more accurate to assess one's heart risk by measuring the levels of apoproteins (the proteins that carry the LDL cholesterol) rather than the LDL itself, but for now the LDL level is still the standard to follow.

- **Keep your HDL cholesterol level above 40 mg/dl if you are a man and above 50 mg/dl if you are a woman.** Women need a higher level of HDL to get the same protective effect. Exercise is the best way to raise the good HDL level. You can also do this through reduction of excess body fat and smoking cessation. Alcohol can raise the level too, but remember not to overdo it. One drink each day for a woman and two drinks for a man—that's the limit. Omega-3 fatty acids can also raise your HDL level and lower your triglyceride level at the same time. You should either eat fatty fish such as salmon three times a week or take fish oil supplements, 2 grams a day, if you are trying to affect your HDL cholesterol level.

- **Keep your triglycerides low.** You want your triglyceride level to be less than 150 mg/dl. A high triglyceride/low HDL ratio is associated with an increased risk of heart disease. Triglycerides are the main form of fat you eat and the main form of fat you store in your body. If triglycerides are high, it is usually a sign of elevated insulin, indicating poor blood sugar control. Tobacco and excessive alcohol consumption also raise triglycerides.

- **Become a lean machine.** Obesity itself is considered an independent risk factor for developing heart disease, particularly if you have a lot of fat accumulation around the waist. Remember that fat cells are not just storage sites. They are very mischievous and secrete more than a hundred different chemicals into your body. Some of these chemicals initiate inflammation, which, as we have just discussed, is at the heart of plaque buildup and heart attacks, so when you allow large fat stores to climb on board, you are asking for trouble.

- **Stay physically active.** A regular exercise program significantly reduces the likelihood of developing heart disease and reduces overall mortality. Even in people who have a history of a prior heart attack, the survival rate increases by 80 percent in those who walk every day for 30 minutes.

- **Maintain a healthy diet.** A heart-healthy diet is high in fruits, vegetables, whole grains, and fish. Minimize red meat and dairy products, which are high in saturated fat. Most of the fat in your diet should be unsaturated. Omega-3 fatty acids are polyunsaturated fats that appear to be particularly healthy for the heart. Foods high in omega-3 fatty acids include fatty fish such as salmon, soybeans, walnuts, and flaxseeds. Moderate alcohol consumption can be considered part of a healthful diet, as I've mentioned before, because it thins the blood, decreases inflammation, and can raise your good HDL cholesterol level. Current research is studying resveratrol, a component of red wine that appears to be a major factor in decreasing inflammation and promoting longevity. The important thing to emphasize here is the word *moderate*. Men should have no more than two drinks a night on average, and women should have no more than one drink a night on average. Too much alcohol will negate these health benefits by creating other health risks, such as breast cancer in women, testicular atrophy in men, and liver disease in both.

- **Develop good stress management skills.** Good stress management is quite important in protecting your heart and blood vessels. Stress is associated with higher rates of heart attacks. People who carry higher amounts of anger and hostility are seven to ten times more likely to die of heart disease. The most important skill when it comes to protecting yourself from the ill effects of stress is to know how well you can flip the switch off and put the stressors out of your mind. If you can flip the switch off easily, you are in good shape.

- **Get a good night's sleep.** This is important for the heart, too. Sleep is important for repairing all of the body's daily wear and tear, as well as for keeping the stress response off and therefore inflammation down. Also, the risk of a heart attack if sleep apnea is present is five to ten times higher than in someone without sleep apnea. Treatment of this disease is therefore critical—be it with weight loss, surgery, or the use of continuous positive airway pressure (CPAP), a treatment where a nasal or oral mask delivers positive pressure to keep the airway open. In some cases, surgery may be indicated.

To sum it up, there are lots of things you can do to prevent heart disease. Lifestyle changes can make a big difference. If you don't know where you stand on some of the risk factors we just talked about, make sure you talk to your doctor to find out. You definitely want to take the reins on this one.

Carlos, a 52-year-old engineer from Tucson, had tried to stop smoking dozens of times but never managed to make it stick. When his brother, only three years older, had a heart attack (and survived), Carlos knew it was time to do something about it. This time he saw his doctor and got medication to reduce his cravings. He started exercising, which not only promoted dopamine production in his brain and helped him break the addiction cycle (see Week 9), it kept him from gaining weight, which had been a problem during his previous attempts. He got rid of all the visual cues around him, such as ashtrays and old cigarette packs, and he stopped going to places where people were smoking. He tried deep breathing and guided imagery whenever he felt stressed, and when he finally kicked the habit, his two sons in their early twenties quit, too. They told him they were proud of him and wanted to be supportive. So Carlos not only improved his own health, he significantly improved the health of his sons as well.

Symptoms of Heart Disease

A heart attack can happen at any time. It is not necessarily linked to physical activity. In fact, the highest incidence of heart attacks is in the early morning.

Classic heart attack symptoms are sudden tightness, squeezing, or pressure over the chest. The pain can radiate up the neck or jaw or down the left arm. Other symptoms can also occur. We call these "associated symptoms." These include sweating, nausea, light-headedness, and shortness of breath. Not all of these symptoms occur; sometimes there's no actual chest pain, just the associated symptoms.

Sometimes the blood vessel doesn't close off so quickly; the process is gradual, with slow plaque buildup. Chest pain in this process is called *angina;* it often occurs during exercise, when your heart demands more blood flow. It can also happen after having an emotional conversation or a big meal. A person will feel the same type of chest tightness or pressure as in a heart attack, but the chest pain will go away in a few minutes once the physical activity is stopped.

Knowing the symptoms of a heart attack or angina is important because acting quickly can save your heart from permanent damage.

Symptoms of a Stroke

A stroke is essentially a "heart attack" of the brain. Usually it occurs because a blood vessel within the brain has become narrowed by plaque and then a clot forms and completely blocks the blood supply. Sometimes it's because a piece of plaque from a bigger artery flicks off and lodges within a smaller brain artery downstream. When a stroke is in progress, people often experience sudden motor loss of one side of the body or numbness. They may have trouble speaking, become confused or clumsy, and sometimes get a headache. In severe cases a person can lose consciousness. If you ever experience these symptoms, the best thing to do is to call 911 and go immediately to the emergency room for rapid evaluation. Time is really of the essence in a stroke, because there is a three-hour window in which medication can be given to successfully break up the clot and restore blood flow. Antiplatelet medications such as aspirin are often given to prevent future strokes or heart attacks because activated platelets promote clotting.

The best treatment for a stroke, though, is prevention—by achieving good control of diabetes, blood pressure, and cholesterol and staying away from tobacco. Lifestyle-related behaviors, such as getting a good night's sleep, managing stress well, exercise and healthy nutrition, also play a critical role. The same things that prevent a heart attack prevent a stroke because the process is really the same. Through lifestyle measures, you can significantly minimize the risks of both heart attack and stroke.

NUTRITION: GOOD FATS, BAD FATS

Now let's take a closer look at fats. Fat is the most misunderstood macronutrient of all. People never seem to know whether fat is universally evil or a good thing to have in their diet. The answer is that *all fats are not created equal.* As you learned earlier, there are good fats and there are bad fats. You may recall that protein and carbohydrate both deliver four calories per gram while fat delivers nine calories per gram. This is true whether the fat is "good" or "bad." So, since fat delivers more calories than protein or carbohydrate, you need to watch your fat intake because either one can quickly bring you to your desired calorie limit.

Fat matters in other ways besides calories, though. Different kinds of fats often promote entirely opposite physiologic consequences in your body. In short, there are two kinds of good fats and two kinds of bad fats. The *good fats* are *unsaturated*—either polyunsaturated or monounsaturated. The *bad fats* are *saturated*—either naturally or through a chemical alteration that creates trans fat. Recent research suggests that saturated fat may not be quite as bad as we had previously thought (although trans fat remains a major villain); however, a healthy diet is still considered to be one that minimizes both saturated and trans fats.

Fat consists of a glycerol backbone to which three fatty acids are attached. The fats vary in the lengths of the fatty acid chains and in the degree of saturation by hydrogen atoms (hydrogenation). Certain fatty acids are considered "essential" to your diet because your body is unable to make them by itself. If you eat a variety of healthful foods, you will be getting enough of these fatty acids.

Fat is essential to the life of all cells. It helps you maintain healthy skin and hair, transport fat-soluble vitamins (A, D, E, and K) throughout your body, and regulate blood cholesterol. Dietary fats also give you a feeling of satiety after a meal because fat slows down the stomach's emptying time. The best-known role of fat is its ability to store the body's extra energy, but it is also quite active; fat deposits secrete more than a hundred different chemicals that can affect your health.

Let's first look at where *bad fats* come from:

- Milk, yogurt, cheese, butter, and sour cream contain saturated fat.

- Animal meat contains saturated fat.

- Processed snack foods and baked foods such as chips, doughnuts, cookies, and crackers usually contain both saturated fat and trans fat although food manufacturers are getting better about taking trans fat out of foods.

- Fast food is usually loaded with trans fat!

- Margarine contains trans fat, except for a few brands such as Smart Beat, Smart Balance, Take Control, and Benecol.

Now let's look at some foods with *good fats:*

- Vegetable oils contain unsaturated fat (except for coconut and palm oil, which contain saturated fat).

- Avocados and olives contain unsaturated fat.

- Fish contain unsaturated fat.

- Nuts and seeds contain unsaturated fat.

- Peanut butter contains unsaturated fat, although most popular brands add a little partially hydrogenated fat so that the oil does not separate out. Natural peanut butter is therefore the healthier choice.

As a rule, anything that comes from an animal contains saturated fat, while anything that comes from plants or fish has mainly unsaturated fat. That's an easy rule of thumb to go by. Also, saturated and trans fats are solid or semisolid at room temperature, while unsaturated fats are liquid at room temperature.

What is trans fat? Trans fat comes from a laboratory where perfectly good unsaturated fat is altered. This process involves adding hydrogen to the bonds in fatty acid chains, thereby saturating many of the previously unsaturated bonds. This factory-made fat became popular because it increased the shelf life of many food products. Unfortunately, we now know that this type of fat is worse for the arteries than saturated fat! It is now mandatory for all food products to announce the presence of trans fat on food labels. If the food has less than .5 gram of trans fat per serving, the fat does not have to be disclosed and will be labeled "0 gram," so it is always a good idea to look at the list of ingredients on the package to see whether "partially hydrogenated vegetable oil" is present. If it is, you are getting trans fat in the food even if the package says you aren't.

The main determinant of whether a fat is good or bad is how it affects your heart, particularly with regard to cholesterol. Polyunsaturated fats lower the bad LDL, so these fats are considered good. Monounsaturated fats not only lower the bad LDL, they also raise the good HDL, so they are considered even better. Olive oil, for example, is a monounsaturated fat. Saturated fats are bad because they raise the bad LDL. Trans fat is even worse because not only does it raise the bad LDL and lower the good HDL, it also makes platelets sticky!

Two special polyunsaturated fats, omega-3 and omega-6, are considered especially heart-healthy because they not only lower the LDL, they also stabilize the heart's rhythm; thin the blood, and decrease inflammation. Omega-6 is plentiful in our food supply, but omega-3 is more limited. As I've already mentioned you can get omega-3 in fatty fish such as salmon, walnuts, canola oil, soybean products, ground flaxseed, or flaxseed oil.

Dietary cholesterol is often included when discussing fats because it shares some characteristics similar to those of fat, but technically it is in the sterol family. Cholesterol is found in the cell membranes of animal tissue and is present in all food from animal sources. There is no cholesterol in plant foods. Your body can survive without getting cholesterol from animal products because your liver can manufacture it. Fats in the diet are modified in the liver to produce different types of cholesterol. For some people, reducing the amount of cholesterol in the diet can reduce the blood cholesterol level. Most people, though, influence their cholesterol level by reducing the amount of saturated fat and trans fat they eat. So remember, if you are working on lowering your cholesterol, yes, you should pay attention to the amount of cholesterol in your diet by getting less than 300 milligrams of dietary cholesterol per day. But reducing the amount of saturated and trans fats in your diet will make the biggest difference of all.

FITNESS: RESISTANCE EXERCISES

Last week you learned why staying strong and stimulating your muscles throughout your life is so important. Now I'd like you to start doing 15 minutes of resistance exercises two or three days each week. Perhaps you can do this strengthening routine on the days that you don't do the extra higher-intensity cardio. Remember to space the sessions out over nonconsecutive days of the week so your muscles have time to recover.

Strength training can benefit everyone. Not only can you improve your ability to function throughout the day, you can also decrease your risk of developing lower-back pain, osteoporosis, hypertension, and diabetes. By performing resistance exercises, you can strengthen your ligaments and tendons and enhance regions of your brain that are responsible for coordination, balance, and general movement skills.

Let's walk through a strength-training workout that you can perform at home or on the road if you travel a lot. All you need is a little space and a resistance band. Resistance bands are readily available online and at sporting goods stores. One band can be purchased for less than ten dollars, and a set of three different-strength bands can be purchased for less than twenty dollars. Bands come in light, medium, and heavy resistance, so you can start at whatever level feels comfortable to you.

In this workout, you will do multijoint exercises that develop total body strength and endurance in a time-efficient manner. Perform each exercise with special attention to form. I suggest that each exercise be performed with 15 repetitions and two sets of each exercise. Allow about 30 seconds' rest after each exercise. If 15 repetitions feel too difficult, start with whatever number of repetitions feels good and slowly work your way up to 15. As your strength increases, you may need to increase the strength of the bands or increase the number of repetitions and sets that you are performing to continue to challenge yourself.

Ideally, strength training is performed after a few minutes of warming up. So take a few minutes to walk or march in place to get your blood pumping!

THE SQUAT

The first exercise is the Squat. Stand with your feet shoulder width apart. Bend your knees as if you are going to sit in a chair and reach back with your buttocks while keeping your chest lifted. This may feel a bit awkward, but if you keep your backside reaching back, your knees will be better protected against undue stress. You do not want your knees to protrude past your toes. Bend only as far as you can safely and with good form. Return to the start position. Do two sets of 15 repetitions. This exercise strengthens the most important muscle in your legs, the quadriceps. The quadriceps is the big muscle in the front of your thigh that is responsible for lifting your body up and lowering it down. A strong quadriceps muscle can help keep your knees and hips healthy, as well as prevent lower-back pain by allowing you to bend from your knees when you need to lift anything.

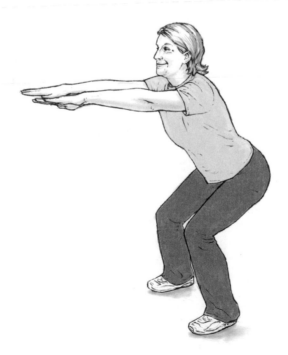

MODIFIED LUNGE

The next exercise works the quadriceps, but it also works the back side of your leg—the gluteal and hamstring muscles. In addition to improving your strength, it improves your balance—an important skill that we don't work on enough as we get older. It's called the Modified Lunge. Stand with your feet in a "stride-step" position. Lower your back knee toward the floor, keeping your chest lifted. Your back heel should automatically lift off the floor. Do not lunge forward over your front foot, and keep your abdomen pulled in. Return to the start position. Do two sets of 15 repetitions for each leg. It's important to keep the gluteal and hamstring muscles strong. They help with posture by supporting the weight you carry in front of your body. The hamstring muscle is also responsible for bending the knee, and general knee movement is important to the knees' overall health.

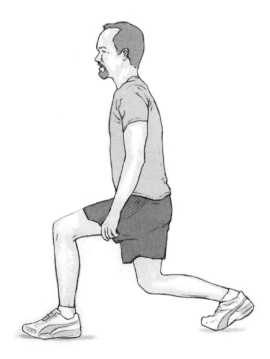

STANDING SINGLE-LEG CALF RAISE

The other major muscle group in the leg is the gastrocnemius, the big calf muscle. This muscle is responsible for raising you onto your tiptoes and putting a spring in your step when you walk fast, jump, or run. One way to strengthen this muscle is with the Standing Single-Leg Calf Raise exercise. Stand with one leg bent, hand resting on a chair or wall. Keeping your chest lifted and tummy in, raise up onto your tiptoe and slowly return to the start position. Keep your weight on your standing leg and resist the urge to transfer your weight onto your front leg. Repeat this same exercise for the other foot as well. Do two sets of 15 repetitions for each foot. Together, the quadriceps, hamstrings, and gastrocnemius form the big-muscle trio that surrounds and supports your knee. If these muscles are strong, they can take some of the excess stress off the bones themselves. They are important to lower-body health and movement, posture, and power.

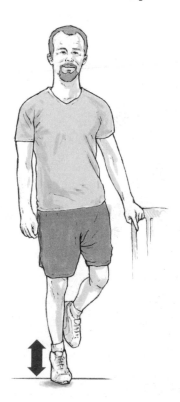

PUSH-UP

Now that you've worked most of the lower-extremity muscles, it's time to turn your attention to the upper body. Let's start with the Modified Push-up. This is a variation on the traditional push-up, which is very difficult to do with good form if you haven't been keeping your upper-body and core strength up. This way you can start this exercise safely, and when you are ready, you can increase the difficulty. Start by facing a desk-height object. Stand about an arm's length away. Place your hands on the edge of the desk, keeping your body straight from the top of your head to your feet. More specifically, tuck in your chin, lift your chest, and keep your abdomen and buttocks tight. Bend your elbows so your chest lowers toward the desk edge—reach with your chest, not with your chin. Push back up to the start position. Do two sets of 15 repetitions. If you need to increase the challenge, use an object with a lower height or perform push-ups on your knees. But remember to keep your form! This exercise strengthens the pectoralis muscle groups, the triceps, and the anterior deltoids. These muscles are important for any sort of pushing activity—such as pushing a heavy door open or pushing yourself out of a chair. Eventually you want to work your way up to a regular push-up (as shown in the illustration), if you can.

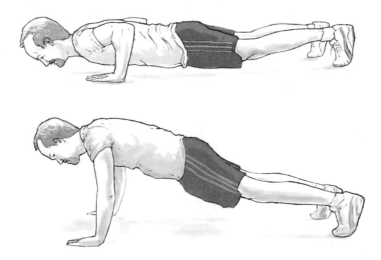

THE ROW

The next exercise is called the Row, and it requires the use of a resistance band. Place the band around a sturdy object at about chest height. If you don't have such an object close by, you can tie a knot in the middle of the band and close a door on it so that the knot is caught in the door frame. Some bands come with an accessory that attaches to the band so you don't need to make the knot. Once you have the band in place, hold on to the handles and back away from the door until your arms are stretched out in front of you and the band is taut but not stretched. From there pull your elbows behind you and squeeze your shoulder blades together. Keep your knees "soft" throughout the exercise. Return to the start position. Do two sets of 15 repetitions. This exercise works the biceps, but, more important, it strengthens the posterior deltoids and rhomboids, the muscles important for good posture. The rhomboids are the muscles in between the shoulder blades. They are responsible for holding you upright and stabilizing the shoulder blades for proper shoulder motion to occur.

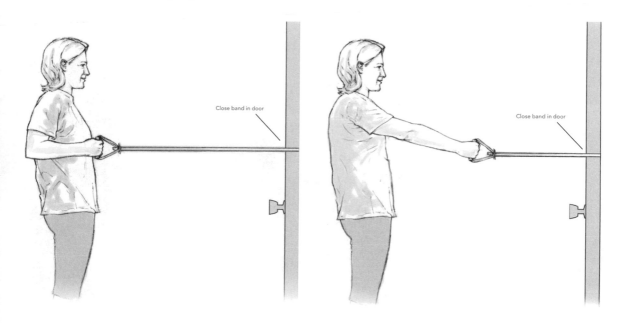

OVERHEAD PRESS

Now let's work our way up to the shoulders. The Overhead Press exercise will do just that. Sit on a sturdy chair on the middle of a resistance band. Make sure you are sitting up straight, with both feet flat on the floor, chin tucked in, and abdomen pulled in. Hold the ends of the band and bring your hands up to shoulder height, with your palms facing forward. Press your hands up to the ceiling and then together by straightening your elbows. Return to the start position. Do two sets of 15 repetitions. Do not perform this exercise if you experience any pain with overhead movement. This exercise strengthens your deltoids (shoulder muscles) and triceps, but with proper form, you can also get the benefit of working your core and postural muscles, like your trapezius muscle group.

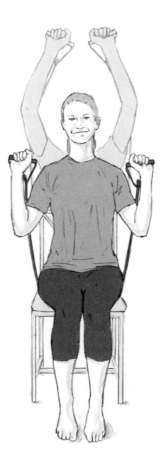

Lat Pull

This exercise will round out your upper-body exercises. It's called the Lat Pull, and it requires the use of a resistance band. To set it up, place the band over a sturdy object overhead. If no such object is available, you can close a door on a knot tied in the middle of the band or use the door accessory included with your band. Hold on to the handles and back away from the door until your elbows are straight and the band is taut but not stretched. At this point, you should be the appropriate distance from the door. You can then sit in a chair or kneel on the ground to get the right angle of pull from the band. Start with your hands overhead and your elbows straight; your body should be bent slightly forward from the hips. Following the angle of the band, pull your elbows out and down, as if you were putting your elbows into your back pockets. Squeeze the bottoms of your shoulder blades together. Slowly return to the start position. Do two sets of 15 repetitions. Whenever you squeeze the shoulder blades together, you want to make sure to keep your abdominal muscles pulled in to avoid arching your lower back. Your latissimus dorsi muscle is the big muscle that runs from your shoulders to your lower back. It is the muscle that creates the V shape in body builders. Now, we're not focusing on turning you into a body builder, but if you can visualize this muscle when you do this exercise, you will enhance your performance of it. And by using your core muscles to stabilize the rest of your body during this exercise, you will work your abdominal and postural muscles, too!

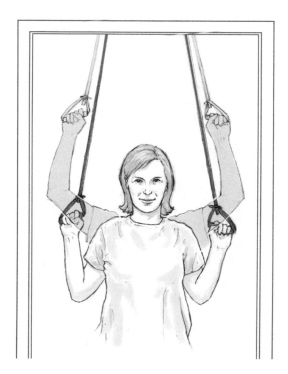

BASIC CRUNCH

The last exercise in your strength-training workout is the Basic Crunch. It is an easy way to work some of your core muscles. Start by lying on your back with your knees bent and your feet flat on the floor. Place your hands behind your head or across your chest, whatever is most comfortable for you. Tuck in your chin and lift your head and the tops of your shoulders off of the ground. During the lift, pull your belly button toward your spine and exhale. Slowly return to the start position. Do two sets of 15 repetitions. It's well known these days how important the abdominal muscles are for posture and for preventing lower-back pain. What is more important is that you remember to use these muscles not just when you exercise but during your daily activities as well. The next time you reach up into a cabinet, try to pull your abdomen in and avoid arching your back. This way, you will be using your core to improve your daily functioning.

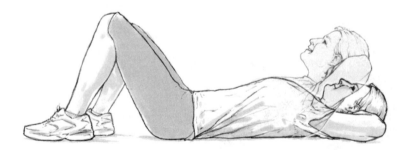

This strength-training workout involves every major muscle group. It is designed to be efficient in both time and energy. Once you are familiar with the exercises, this routine should take you 15 to 20 minutes from start to finish. Perform this routine two to three days a week, and it will enhance your life with better strength and function. Remember to rest 30 seconds between sets.

RESISTANCE EXERCISES: A QUICK REVIEW

The Squat	2 sets of 15 repetitions
Modified Lunge	2 sets of 15 repetitions on each leg
Standing Single-Leg Calf Raise	2 sets of 15 repetitions on each foot
Push-up	2 sets of 15 repetitions
The Row*	2 sets of 15 repetitions
Overhead Press*	2 sets of 15 repetitions
Lat Pull*	2 sets of 15 repetitions
Basic Crunch	2 sets of 15 repetitions

*Requires a resistance band.

LEARN IT!

- Heart disease is the leading cause of death in the United States; most of its risk factors can be prevented or modified through lifestyle changes.

- The risk factors for heart disease that can be eliminated or improved are:

  - Smoking

  - High LDL cholesterol level

  - High blood pressure

  - High blood sugar level

  - Stress

  - Sleep deprivation

- 75 percent of heart attacks are caused by arterial plaque rupture in your arteries.

- Vital Statistics:

  ▸ **Blood pressure** should be 130/80 mm/Hg or less.

  ▸ **Blood sugar** should be less than 100 mg/dl, fasting (no food or drink, except water, for twelve hours prior to testing).

  ▸ **LDL cholesterol** should be less than 130 mg/dl in everyone, fasting (no food or drink, except water, for twelve hours prior to testing).

  ▸ **HDL cholesterol** should be above 40 mg/dl for men and above 50 mg/dl for women.

  ▸ **Triglycerides** should be less than 150 mg/dl, fasting (no food or drink, except water, for twelve hours prior to testing).

- Most cholesterol is made in your liver. The cholesterol in your diet affects only 10 percent of the cholesterol in your bloodstream. Cholesterol is made largely from the saturated and trans fats in your diet.

- Exercise is the best way to raise your good HDL cholesterol level.

- All fats are not created equal.

  ▸ **Best:** Monounsaturated fats lower bad LDL and raise good HDL levels.

  ▸ **Better:** Polyunsaturated fats lower the bad LDL level.

  ▸ **Bad:** Saturated fats raise the bad LDL level.

  ▸ **Terrible:** Trans fats raise bad LDL and lower good HDL levels.

- Saturated fats come from animals and are solid or semisolid at room temperature.

- Unsaturated fats come from plants and fish and are liquid at room temperature.

PERSONALIZE IT!

This week, work on your Unique Brain.

No two brains are the same. Everyone is born with a unique DNA blueprint, and everyone has different life experiences. So although the basic principles for staying healthy are the same for everyone, you need to learn how to make these principles work for you in your own life.

Here are some examples of how people in The Program have personalized this brain principle and put it into action.

- **Challenge:** How can you eat healthfully when you come home exhausted at the end of each day and don't feel like cooking?

  - Anastasia W., a 32-year-old teacher, loved to cook, so she cooked on weekends and stored meals to eat on weekdays. This provided her with easy, healthful meals she could pull out when she got home tired at the end of the day.

  - Lisa T., a 42-year-old mother of one, hated to cook. In order to eat healthfully, Lisa stopped by the gourmet grocery market each day and bought marinated fish or chicken and already prepared vegetables that she then brought home and grilled.

  - Jane W., a 40-year-old mother of four, organized a group of friends who rotated weeknights for cooking. They each took turns one night of the week making one big, healthy meal, and then distributed it to all of the group members' homes. Then they sat back for the rest of the week and enjoyed having home-cooked meals delivered to them!

- **Challenge:** What's the best way of tracking your food intake?

  - Molly U., 50 years old, loved to track her food and exercise on spreadsheets. She liked keeping track of her food servings and calories.

▸ Jerry P., a 39-year-old salesman, preferred keeping an index card in his pocket, and he simply wrote down what he ate at the time he ate it.

▸ Jim K., a 36-year-old computer consultant, did not even want to write anything down. He took pictures of his meals with his cell phone and kept a picture food log on his computer to keep himself accountable.

LIVE IT!

▪ Review last week's goals and create this week's short-term goals. Remember to create strategies around your obstacles that will work for you in your own unique life.

▪ List your risk factors for heart disease. Decide which ones you would like to modify. If you smoke, talk to your doctor about strategies and medications now available to help you quit.

▪ Identify the types of fat in your diet this week. Are you eating mostly unsaturated fats or saturated and trans fats?

▪ Incorporate 15 minutes of resistance exercises into your exercise routine two to three times each week.

DIMINISHING DIABETES

We can do anything we want to do if we stick to it long enough.

—HELEN KELLER

RIGHT NOW, WE ARE in the middle of a worldwide epidemic—of type 2 diabetes. Some of you may think, "Oh, I don't need to worry, there's no diabetes in my family," but everyone needs to work to prevent this disease, regardless of your family history. Almost ten percent of the U.S. population has type 2 diabetes, and 20 percent of those over the age of 65 have type 2 diabetes. What's really troubling is that the number of diabetics in this country is expected to double by the year 2025!

Diabetes is a condition in which you have a higher-than-normal blood sugar level (also called blood glucose level) in your bloodstream. You are diagnosed as having diabetes if your blood sugar level is over 125 mg/dl after you have been without food for twelve hours. You are diagnosed as having prediabetes if your blood sugar range is 100 to 125 mg/dl. An elevated blood sugar level is harmful to all of the arteries in your body, so over time, if your blood sugar level remains elevated, the organs in your body will start to malfunction and die. This can lead to heart attacks, strokes, kidney failure, and blindness. A high blood sugar level is also toxic to your nerves and immune cells, and can cause painful, numb extremities, bowel and bladder problems, difficulty with erections if you are a man, poor wound healing, and frequent infections.

> **Diabetes**: Your fasting blood sugar level is over 125 mg/dl.
>
> **Prediabetes**: Your fasting blood sugar level is between 100 and 125 mg/dl.

Here's how it all works. You eat a carbohydrate. The carbohydrate is broken down into glucose. Glucose is a simple sugar. In fact, any macronutrient (protein, carbohydrate, or fat) can be broken down into a glucose by-product—carbohydrates are just the easiest to break down into glucose because a carbohydrate is really just one long glucose string. The glucose is then absorbed and carried to all your cells by your bloodstream.

Diabetes

24 million Americans have diabetes. 90 to 95 percent of diabetics have type 2 diabetes.

There is an organ in your body that is called the pancreas that is acutely aware of your blood sugar level. When your pancreas senses sugar, it responds by secreting insulin. Insulin goes to every cell in your body and attaches to insulin receptors. It's like a key fitting into a lock. Once the insulin attaches to the receptor, glucose is allowed to enter into the cell.

If glucose can't enter the cell, it builds up in the blood and becomes toxic. In addition to this, if a cell doesn't sense enough glucose coming into it, it will scream at the pancreas to produce more insulin. It will have a chemical temper tantrum because the cells need glucose to sustain not just their life but your life as well. This important reaction is pretty simple. Glucose combines with oxygen inside the cell to produce adenosine triphosphate (ATP). ATP is an energy storage unit. You can think of ATP as a battery. It supplies the energy

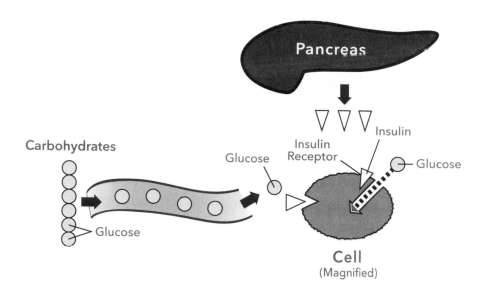

Pancreas

Insulin

Carbohydrates

Glucose

Insulin
Receptor

Glucose

Glucose

Cell
(Magnified)

(Diagram not to scale)

to drive all the reactions in your body so that you can live. When your cells don't get the glucose they need to make the energy juice ATP, it's just like what happens to your car when the battery dies: it won't start.

Occasionally, our bodies get confused and our immune system attacks our own organs. This is what happens in type 1 diabetes. In type 1 diabetes the body makes proteins that attack one's own pancreas. That's a big deal. Without a functioning pancreas, a person cannot live unless given an alternative supply of insulin.

Type 2 diabetes is a different condition. Here, the problem lies largely with the insulin receptors. With type 2 diabetes, the pancreas often starts out just fine. It can produce as much insulin as it wants, but the insulin receptors have become less sensitive. They don't work as well, so glucose has a harder time getting into the cells. Then the cells start to scream and the pancreas pumps out more insulin and floods the receptors so that sugar (glucose) can eventually enter the cells.

Prediabetes
57 million Americans have prediabetes.

This works for a little while. The cells gets their sugar, so they're happy, and the pancreas seems to do fine, at least in the short run, by producing larger amounts of insulin. But there's a catch. The high insulin levels actually harm you in three important ways.

First, the insulin can cause your blood pressure to rise and you can develop high blood pressure. Second, the insulin can adversely affect your cholesterol profile. It raises your triglyceride level and it lowers your good, protective HDL cholesterol level. Finally—and this is a pretty dirty trick—the insulin goes to your fat cells and promotes fat deposits, especially in the area around the waist, giving you an apple-shaped body that is particularly bad for your heart.

Good News

In a large prevention study for people at high risk for developing type 2 diabetes, small changes in lifestyle over three years reduced the risk by 58 percent, and for people over 70 the risk went down by 71 percent.

Why do fat cells get fatter because of high doses of insulin? All cells have insulin receptors. But for some reason, the fat cells remain sensitive to insulin, even when the muscle cells become more resistant. So the sugar is preferentially let into the fat cells rather than the muscle cells. Once inside the fat cells, the sugar is not used for creating ATP; instead, it is just used to store fat. This is handy if starvation is right around the corner (as it often was for our prehistoric ancestors), but for most people today, this is an issue. The real zinger here is that fat cells secrete a chemical that encourages the muscles' insulin receptors to become less sensitive. That means the pancreas has to churn out more insulin (which the fat cells grab), the fat cells become even fatter and secrete more of their chemicals, and the vicious cycle continues.

Now that you understand this process, you can see how important it is to keep your insulin receptors as sensitive as possible throughout your entire life. This is crucial for staying healthy and aging well, not just for preventing diabetes. So how can you influence this process? It turns out that there are five main factors that control insulin sensitivity.

First, there is a **genetic contribution.** You can't change your genes, but fortunately genetics are only one part of the story, and not even the most important part. If you have a family history of type 2 diabetes, you probably aren't starting out with the most sensitive of insulin receptors in the first place. That means it is especially important that you do everything you can to influence the sensitivity of your insulin receptors.

Aging also affects your insulin receptors; the older we get, the less sticky our insulin receptors tend to be.

So far, I've told you about two things that affect your insulin receptors that are not under your control, but now I'll tell you about three things you can do to optimize the sensitivity of your insulin receptors.

1   **Be a lean machine.** As I just discussed, the more fat you have on your body, the more your fat cells will secrete chemicals that directly sabotage your muscle cells' ability to use insulin; this will cause your insulin level to rise, promoting further fat deposition. Losing excess weight will lower both your insulin level and your blood sugar level. This will also allow you to lose weight more easily in the future should you need to.

2   **Exercise on a regular basis.** Exercise improves the sensitivity of the insulin receptors. It stimulates the release of growth factors, one of which is insulinlike growth factor–1 (IGF-1), that help your insulin attach to the insulin receptors and that stimulate the production of even more insulin receptors. So doing more exercise will lower both your insulin level and blood sugar level, bringing them closer to normal.

3   **Eat high-fiber, unprocessed complex carbohydrates combined with protein.** Avoid processed, refined low-fiber carbohydrates. Your insulin receptors work best if you keep your blood sugar level in a steady, even range. To do this, you need to avoid processed foods that have been

broken down so much that your body digests them too easily, because this allows your body to absorb sugar too rapidly. To keep your blood sugar level nice and steady, your carbohydrates should come from high-fiber whole grains, fruits, and vegetables. These foods are more difficult to break down, so they are absorbed in a slower, more gradual fashion. Eating a little protein and fat at each meal will also keep your blood sugar from rising and dropping too quickly because your body will experience a more gradual, lasting elevation in blood sugar.

The message here is not new: eat right, exercise, and maintain a healthy body weight. But now that you understand the process, it might be easier to see why these guidelines are so important.

For Those Who Have Diabetes

I know it takes a lot of work to control your blood sugar on a daily basis, and you're not alone if you sometimes feel discouraged. It is worth the effort, though.

As a diabetic, you are no doubt familiar with the hemoglobin A1c (HgbA1c) test, but do you know exactly what it measures? The sugar in one's blood tends to attach to proteins, so one way of measuring your average blood sugar over the past three months is to measure the amount of sugar attached to your hemoglobin. Hemoglobin is a protein that carries oxygen in the red blood cells circulating through your body. Normal blood sugar ranges are associated with a certain level of sugar bonding to the hemoglobin (measured as HgbA1c, which is normally below 6 mg/dl), but large amounts indicate chronically elevated blood sugar and a higher risk of diabetic complications. For those with HgbA1c above 7 mg/dl, a 1 percent drop can translate into a one-third reduction in diabetic complications. That's a one-third reduction for *every* 1 percent drop in HgbA1c. That's huge! Also, better blood sugar control can help you feel better on a day-to-day basis by giving you higher energy levels and fewer mood fluctuations. It is so worth going the extra mile on this one. Even small reductions in your blood sugar can make a big difference in diabetes.

When you have diabetes, it can be hard to keep track of all the things you're supposed to do for your health. Here's a simple way of remembering. It's called the "ABCs and double-DEFs" of diabetes. Let's go over what this means.

A is for **hemoglobin A1c,** the measure of your average blood sugar level over the previous three months. This should be checked two to four times a year. Your goal for hemoglobin A1c is less than 7 mg/dl.

B is for **blood pressure.** Your blood pressure should be checked at every doctor's visit, but it is also a good idea to have a blood pressure monitor at home so you can check it yourself. Aim for a blood pressure of less than 130/80; the lower, the better.

C is for **cholesterol.** Your cholesterol should be checked one to two times a year. Your LDL goal, since you have diabetes, is less than 100 mg/dl (less than 70 mg/dl if you also have heart disease).

DD is for proper **dental care** and a healthy **diet.** Your diet for diabetes is no different from simply following a healthy diet. Whole grains, fruits and vegetables, lean meat, unsaturated fat—you've heard it before. Everyone should be eating this way. We should all cut back on sweets because sugar from pure sweets, treats, and refined foods is absorbed too rapidly, and when you have diabetes you are particularly vulnerable to sugar swings. Nonetheless, there is intrinsically no difference in the way you should eat if you have diabetes and the way you should eat to achieve optimal health. With diabetes it is especially important to keep your teeth and gums healthy. Flossing helps stimulate the blood flow to your gums to keep them healthy; this is particularly important in diabetes because a high blood sugar level can promote plaque buildup in the tiny end arteries that feed the gums.

EE is for a yearly **eye exam** and regular **exercise.** It is important to have your eyes checked on a regular basis since the blood flow in the back of the eyes (necessary for sight) can be reduced in diabetes; however, this is very treatable when caught early. Exercise is important since it improves sensitivity to insulin and helps keep excess weight off.

FF is for **feet checks** and **flu vaccine.** Check your feet every night before you go to bed, as they can develop sores due to the reduction in blood flow and your compromised immune system. In addition, all diabetics are strongly encouraged to get a yearly flu inoculation (as well as the pneumococcal vaccine that protects against a certain type of bacterial pneumonia) because high blood sugar levels impair the immune system, allowing infections to occur more easily.

Following the ABCs and double-DEFs of diabetes will go a long way to keep you optimally healthy. The good news is that with diabetes you can have a lot of control over the course of your health.

Cathy, a 48-year-old business consultant from Toledo, was a type 2 diabetic who was on maximum oral medications when her doctor told her she was going to need to start insulin injections. Her doctor said that her blood sugar was just too poorly controlled for her to continue as she was. Cathy made up her mind to lose 35 pounds. She cut out sweets and alcohol and began to exercise regularly. Before long, she had lost 30 pounds and her fasting blood sugar level had dropped from 200 to 126 mg/dl! Not only was she able to avoid starting insulin injections, she was even able to discontinue two of her other medications!

NUTRITION: GOOD CARBS, BAD CARBS

Carbohydrates make up about half of the daily calories in the typical American diet. Carbohydrates are the most common worldwide source of calories because they are readily accessible and cheap. Carbohydrates include all the sugars, starch, and fiber we eat. Sugars and starch are the body's most efficient fuel because they can easily be broken down into glucose to produce almost instant energy. Fiber, however, has no calories because it is not absorbed by the digestive system.

WHAT FOODS CONTAIN CARBOHYDRATES?

- Grains such as breads, cereals, rice, and pasta

- Vegetables

- Fruits

- Milk and yogurt

- Most desserts, sodas, and snack foods

- Most meat substitutes such as beans, lentils, and tofu

It is important to recognize that foods that are composed mainly of carbohydrates may also contain protein and fat. Breads, for example, contain a little protein and fat in addition to carbohydrates, but milk, yogurt, beans, and lentils contain much higher amounts of protein. Tofu is made from soybeans and so is high in protein. While some dairy products such as milk and yogurt contain carbohydrates, others such as cheese and butter do not. Cheese is all fat and protein; butter is pure fat.

There are two general types of carbohydrates: simple (sugars) and complex (starches and fiber). Simple carbohydrates are one, two, or at most three units of sugar linked together. Simple carbohydrates that contain only one sugar unit are *monosaccharides* and include glucose (sometimes called dextrose), fructose, and galactose. Monosaccharides are seldom found free in nature. They are generally linked together and bonded into what is known as a *disaccharide*. Sucrose is a disaccharide made from glucose combining with fructose. Food sources of sucrose are fruit, vegetables, honey, table sugar, sugarcane, maple syrup, and maple sugar. Lactose is a disaccharide made from glucose combining with galactose. This is the principal sugar in milk. People with lactose intolerance have trouble breaking the bond between glucose and galactose; therefore their small intestine does not easily absorb it. Those with lactose intolerance may experience bloating, abdominal cramps, and diarrhea when consuming large amounts of dairy products. Three quarters of the world's population has some degree of lactose intolerance. Maltose is a disaccharide made of two glucoses linked together. It is found in malt products and some breakfast cereals.

The body doesn't have to work very hard to break down sugars and convert them into a quick burst of energy. Common simple sugars include table sugar,

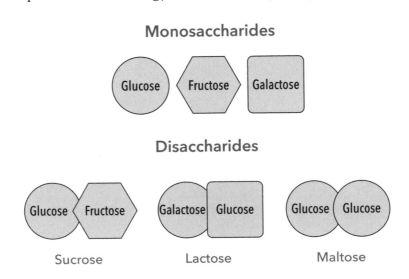

Monosaccharides

Glucose Fructose Galactose

Disaccharides

Glucose Fructose
Sucrose

Galactose Glucose
Lactose

Glucose Glucose
Maltose

jam, jelly, syrup, fruit juice, and honey. In addition, many Americans consume quite a lot of sugar in processed foods such as sodas, cakes, pies, and cookies. Simple sugars can pose a threat to your health when consumed in large amounts. Common chronic health problems such as diabetes, heart disease, and obesity are often the result of a diet rich in simple sugars.

Complex carbohydrates are long chains of glucose (sugar) units that form starch and indigestible fiber. Complex carbohydrates occur in all plant foods. Fruits, vegetables, and whole grains are excellent sources of complex carbohydrates that contain both starch and fiber. In contrast to simple carbohydrates, starches are broken down slowly, especially if the starch is in its whole form and not processed or refined. As mentioned before, in the typical American diet, 50 percent of the calories come from carbohydrates. Unfortunately, at least half of the carbohydrates in a typical American diet are in the form of simple sugars and refined carbohydrates.

Refined foods are also usually stripped of fiber. Fibers are complex carbohydrates that cannot be digested or absorbed. Fiber has no calories but provides lots of health benefits. Although starch can be broken down and absorbed, the presence of fiber slows down its absorption process, resulting in a steadier blood sugar level. Maintaining a steady blood sugar level protects against the effects of insulin that contribute to diabetes, heart disease, high blood pressure, elevated triglycerides, decreased HDL cholesterol, and weight gain.

Fiber is also a friend to your gastrointestinal tract, moving food through the system and thus reducing constipation and your risk of colon cancer. The less straining a person does during bowel movements, the less likely he or she is to develop conditions such as diverticulosis or hemorrhoids. Fiber also forms a mesh in the gut that promotes the growth of healthy bacteria that aid in digestion and immune protection.

The human body is designed for fiber. We need it. *The recommended daily amount of fiber is 25 to 35 grams.* The typical American diet contains 11 grams.

FIBER CONTENT OF FOODS

FOOD ITEM	SERVING SIZE	FIBER (GRAMS)
GRAINS		
BREADS		
Waffle, Kashi	1	3.0
Tortillas, corn	2	3.0
Bread, pita, whole wheat	1/2 large	2.3
Bread, whole wheat	1 slice	1.9
Bread, rye	1 slice	1.8
Bagel	1 ounce	0.7
Bread, white	1 slice	0.7
English muffin, white flour	1/2	0.5
CEREALS		
Fiber One	3/4 cup	21.0
All-Bran	1/2 cup	10.0
Kashi, Heart to Heart Honey Toasted Oat	3/4 cup	5.0
Barbara's Bakery Puffins Original	3/4 cup	5.0
Raisin Bran	1/2 cup	3.5
Cheerios	1 cup	3.0
Grape-Nuts	1/4 cup	3.0
Quaker Instant Oatmeal	1 packet	3.0
Total	3/4 cup	3.0
Wheat germ	3 tablespoons	3.0
Wheaties	3/4 cup	3.0
Granola, low-fat	1/4 cup	1.5
Special K	1 cup	0.9
Rice Krispies	1 cup	0.3

FOOD ITEM	SERVING SIZE	FIBER (GRAMS)
CRACKERS		
Triscuit, Original	4 pieces	2.2
Graham cracker square	2 pieces	2.0
Kashi TLC, Original 7 Grain	10 pieces	1.3
Rice cakes	2 large	0.8
Wheat Thins	8 pieces	0.5
Ritz	5 pieces	0.0
OTHER		
Spaghetti, whole wheat	1/2 cup, cooked	3.1
Sweet potato, baked	1/2 cup	2.9
Potato, baked	1/2	1.9
Rice, brown, long grain	1/2 cup, cooked	1.7
Spaghetti, white	1/2 cup, cooked	1.3
Couscous	1/2 cup, cooked	1.1
Rice, white, long grain	1/2 cup, cooked	0.3
SNACK FOODS		
Popcorn, air-popped	3 cups	3.6
Fig Newton	2 pieces	1.0
Pretzels, salted classic thin style	8	1.0
VEGETABLES		
Beets	1 cup, canned	3.1
Carrots	1 cup, raw	3.1
Asparagus	1 cup, raw	2.8
Eggplant	1 cup, raw	2.8
Onion	1 cup, raw	2.7
Cauliflower	1 cup, raw	2.5
Peppers, green, yellow, red	1 cup, raw	2.5

FOOD ITEM	SERVING SIZE	FIBER (GRAMS)
Broccoli	1 cup, raw	2.4
Turnips	1 cup, raw	2.3
Tomato	1 cup, raw	2.2
Okra	1/2 cup, cooked	2.0
Brussels sprouts	1/2 cup, cooked	2.0
Mushrooms	1/2 cup, canned	1.9
Radishes	1 cup, raw	1.9
Cabbage	1 cup, raw	1.8
Tomato sauce, no salt added	1/2 cup	1.8
Celery	1 cup	1.6
Zucchini	1 cup, raw	1.4
Mushrooms	1 cup, raw	1.3
Squash	1 cup, raw	1.2
Lettuce, romaine	1 cup, raw	1.0
Tomato and vegetable juice, low sodium	1/2 cup	0.9
Cucumber	1 cup	0.8
Spinach	1 cup, raw	0.7
FRUITS		
Raspberries	1 cup	8.0
Blackberries	1 cup	7.6
Pear	1 large	4.4
Apple	1 large	3.7
Blueberries	1 cup	3.6
Orange	1 large	3.6
Strawberries	1 cup	3.3
Kiwi	1 large	2.7

FOOD ITEM	SERVING SIZE	FIBER (GRAMS)
Nectarine	1 large	2.7
Banana	1 small	2.6
Peach	1 large	2.6
Cherries	1 cup	2.5
Grapefruit	1 cup sections	2.5
Figs	3 dried	2.5
Mandarin orange	1 large	2.2
Pineapple, fresh	1 cup	2.2
Apricots	3 raw	2.1
Dates	3	2.0
Figs	1 raw	1.9
Plums	2 raw	1.8
Apricots	1/4 cup, dried	1.6
Applesauce	1/2 cup	1.5
Cantaloupe	1 cup	1.4
Honeydew melon	1 cup	1.4
Fruit cocktail	1/2 cup	1.2
Grapes	1 cup	0.6
Watermelon	1 cup, cubed	0.6
FRUIT JUICE		
Prune	1/2 cup	1.3
Grapefruit	1/2 cup	0.0
MEAT SUBSTITUTES		
Lentils	1/2 cup	8.2
Kidney beans	1/2 cup	8.2
Pinto beans	1/2 cup	7.7

FOOD ITEM	SERVING SIZE	FIBER (GRAMS)
Black beans	1/2 cup	7.5
Refried beans	1/2 cup	6.7
Chickpeas	1/2 cup	6.2
Nuts, almonds, unsalted	1 ounce	3.3
Sunflower seeds, unsalted	1 ounce	3.0
Tofu	4 ounces or 1/2 cup	2.9
Nuts, mixed, unsalted	1 ounce	2.6
Peanut butter	2 tablespoons	1.9
Egg with yolk	2 large	0.0
Egg, white	1 large	0.0

DAIRY

Cheddar cheese	1 ounce	0.0
Cottage cheese, 1%	4 ounces	0.0
Milk, nonfat	1 cup	0.0
Yogurt, Dannon Light & Fit	1 container	0.0
Yogurt, Yoplait Light	1 container	0.0

MEATS

BEEF

Beef, ground, 95% lean	3 ounces, cooked	0.0
Beef, top sirloin	3 ounces, cooked	0.0

FISH

Halibut	3 ounces, cooked	0.0
Salmon	3 ounces, cooked	0.0
Snapper	3 ounces, cooked	0.0
Sole	3 ounces, cooked	0.0
Swordfish	3 ounces, cooked	0.0
Tuna, in water	3 ounces	0.0

FOOD ITEM	SERVING SIZE	FIBER (GRAMS)
POULTRY		
Chicken, breast	3 ounces, cooked	0.0
Turkey, breast, sliced	3 ounces, cooked	0.0
FATS		
MONOUNSATURATED FATS		
Hummus	2 tablespoons	1.7
Avocado	2 tablespoons	1.2
Peanuts, unsalted	10	0.5
Almonds, unsalted	7	0.4
Canola oil	1 teaspoon	0.0
Guacamole	1 tablespoon	0.0
Olive oil	1 teaspoon	0.0

Nutrient information obtained from individual food companies and www.nal.usda.gov/fnic/foodcomp/search.

A QUICK RULE OF THUMB

- Whole-grain products have 2 to 5 grams (or more) of fiber per serving.

- Vegetables have 2 to 3 grams of fiber per serving.

- Fruits have 2 to 4 grams of fiber per serving.

- Beans have 5 to 8 grams of fiber per serving.

Tally up the total daily fiber grams you consume on a typical day. Where are they coming from? Look at the fiber grams in the "Fiber Content of Foods" table. If you are not already eating an average of 25 to 35 grams of fiber per day, how can you restructure your daily meal planning so that this is possible? Could you add a high-fiber cereal in the morning? Do you want to add a fiber supplement to your meals? Can you switch your grains to whole grains from refined? Can you commit to getting your recommended quota of fruits and vegetables?

EASY DOES IT

Increase the fiber in your diet slowly. Sudden adoption of a high-fiber diet can cause abdominal discomfort, including gas and diarrhea. Increase your intake of fiber gradually over several weeks to avoid these problems.

TIPS FOR CHOOSING HEALTHY CARBOHYDRATES

- Begin your day with a high-fiber cereal; aim for 5 grams of fiber per serving. Look for high-fiber cereal brands such as Kashi, Healthy Valley, or Nature's Path.

- Eat at least five servings of fruits and vegetables per day. Keep freshly cut, ready-to-eat vegetables and fruits in the refrigerator to eat for snacks.

- Throw vegetables into your food while cooking dinner to bulk it up.

- Eat whole fruit instead of fruit juice. You'll get fiber and more nutrients this way. Whole fruit also fills you up more than the equivalent number of calories in a liquid form.

- Blend fruit and nonfat yogurt in a blender for a healthy breakfast or snack.

- Eat whole-grain breads instead of processed, refined breads. These breads should list whole wheat, whole-wheat flour, or another whole grain as the first ingredient on the food label. Aim for brands that have at least 2 grams of fiber per serving.

- Replace all-purpose flour in recipes with whole-grain flour.

- Replace white pasta with whole-wheat pasta.

- Say good-bye to white rice and hello to brown rice.

- Add barley to soups and stews.

- Add cooked bulgur wheat to salads, stews, and casseroles.

- Add wheat germ to yogurt or cereal.

- Add crushed bran cereal or unprocessed wheat bran to baked products such as breads, muffins, or casseroles, roughly one tablespoon per serving. You can also use bran products as crunchy toppings for salads, yogurt, or uncooked vegetables.

- Add dried fruit to oatmeal, cereal, muffins, and yogurt.

- Eat more beans, peas, and lentils. You can add them to salads, soups, and side dishes.

- Enjoy low-fat popcorn.

It is important to shift the balance of carbohydrates away from simple sugars and refined carbohydrates and toward unprocessed carbohydrates, such as whole grains, fruits, and vegetables.

FITNESS: WHY BE FLEXIBLE?

This week I'm going to talk about flexibility. Muscles are attached to bones with tendons. Some people are born with very pliable tendons. Those people are flexible. Over time, though, everyone's tendons start to lose their pliability and become stiff. Inactivity also leads to stiffness. Gentle stretching encourages your muscles and tendons to become more pliable.

Increasing the flexibility in your muscles, tendons, and connective tissues is much like stretching a rubber band. If you stretch a rubber band and then let it go, it will return to its original length, but if you keep it stretched long enough, it will remain a slightly longer length.

Why should you care? One reason is that day-to-day activities are simply easier and less painful if you aren't stiff. Also, if you are a competitive athlete, some sports require flexibility to generate enough force from the muscles to allow jumping or cutting movements. Some of these sports include volleyball, basketball, soccer, and tennis.

Proper nutrition plays a role in flexibility because the body depends on being able to make certain substances that are important to the elasticity of connective tissue. Also, if you have poor blood sugar control, you may eventually develop inadequate blood flow to the tendons, which can lead to recurrent tendonitis. This is often seen in poorly controlled diabetics.

Hydration is also important. The water content of connective tissue decreases with aging and contributes to stiffness. The water content also decreases with inactivity. An example of this can be seen in someone who has just had a cast or splint removed. Two weeks of immobilization can cause the hydration of connective tissue to decrease by up to 50 percent, creating a stiff and often achy joint.

Too much physical or emotional stress can decrease flexibility because muscles tense when the sympathetic nervous system fires. The same thing occurs with inadequate sleep.

Nutrition, activity, sleep, stress management—they all play a role in your body's flexibility, just as they do in your overall health. Next week, I'll introduce a simple stretching routine you can easily do at home in a few minutes' time. Improvement in flexibility happens pretty quickly, so stretching can be quite a satisfying part of your routine.

LEARN IT!

- **Diabetes:** diagnosis given when the fasting blood sugar is over 125 mg/dl.

- **Prediabetes:** diagnosis given when the fasting blood sugar level is between 100 and 125 mg/dl.

- **Type 1 diabetes** occurs when the body's antibodies attack the pancreas, thus destroying its ability to produce insulin.

- **Type 2 diabetes** occurs when the body's insulin receptors become less sensitive.

- **You can dramatically reduce your risk factors for diabetes by:**

  - Losing excess body weight.

  - Exercising regularly.

  - Eating high-fiber, unprocessed carbohydrates.

  - Avoiding simple sugars and refined carbohydrates.

- **There are two types of carbohydrates:**

  - Simple (sugars)

  - Complex (starch and fiber)

- **Carbohydrates occur in plant food** but are also found in some dairy products such as milk and yogurt.

- **Fiber is found in plant products, not animal products.**

- **Recommended daily fiber intake: 25 to 35 grams a day.**

- **Regularly stretching increases one's flexibility.**

PERSONALIZE IT!

This week, work on your Rational Brain.

The human brain, specifically your frontal cortex, is highly developed for problem solving. You can use this problem-solving talent to strategize around the various challenges that come up when you are trying to practice healthful habits. You can also use your frontal cortex to better understand why you behave the way you do, and then you can consciously work to substitute healthful behaviors for unhealthful ones. Finally, you can use your Rational Brain to connect back to your Emotional Brain to modulate your mood or stress level.

Here are some examples of how people in The Program have personalized this brain principle and put it into action.

- Rachel F., a 32-year-old new mother who also worked as a full-time editor, had very little time to include exercise in her life. She worked all day and could not bear to be away from her baby a moment longer to exercise when she came home from work. So Rachel's mother (who watched the baby during the day) met her with the baby in her stroller at the train station at the end of each day and Rachel walked home with the baby, a two-mile distance, instead of having her mother drive them home. This provided time for Rachel to be with her baby, get exercise, and make the transition from her fast-paced work life to a more relaxed time at home with her husband and baby.

- Mary C., a 35-year-old schoolteacher, had trouble controlling how much she ate when she came home from work every day because she was really hungry. She solved this problem by keeping healthy, nonperishable snacks in her purse and desk at all times so she never reached the dinner hour feeling famished.

- Andrew T., a 44-year-old marketing executive, found that work always seemed to edge out the time he had planned for exercise. He decided to bring walking shoes to work and started to take walks at lunch. If he happened to have a lunch meeting that pulled him off his schedule, he tried to arrange a different time to walk, even scheduling meetings with work colleagues where they could talk while they walked.

- Eric B., a 61-year-old research scientist, put an exercise bike in his office so that he could take frequent exercise breaks to brainstorm about problems he was having in his lab experiments.

LIVE IT!

- Review last week's goals and create this week's short-term goals.

- List your risk factors for diabetes and decide which ones you want to work on.

- Identify the types of carbohydrates in your diet. Are there any refined or processed carbohydrates you are willing to give up or at least cut back on?

- Track your daily fiber grams this week. Are you getting 25 to 35 grams each day?

THE SLEEP CURE

To accomplish great things, we must not only act but also dream, not only plan but also believe.

—ANATOLE FRANCE

WE'VE TALKED ABOUT HOW nutrition, fitness, and stress all fit into the big picture of your health. Now I'd like to teach you about sleep and why it's so important. We need sleep to feel refreshed and alert, but we also need it to reduce the risk of becoming obese and developing high blood pressure, diabetes, heart disease, infections, and even cancer. How can sleep have so much of an impact on our health?

Let's review what happens during sleep. There are two categories of sleep: non-REM and REM. Non-REM sleep makes up 75 percent of a normal sleep period. It is divided into four stages called stages one, two, three, and four. Each stage brings on progressively deeper sleep. Non-REM sleep is an essential time for your body to repair. During non-REM sleep, your brain is fairly quiet but your body tends to move more. Growth hormone is secreted during non-REM sleep, and this promotes muscle repair and stimulates tissue growth. Interleukins are also released in high amounts. They stimulate your immune system so you stay strong in fighting off infections, and they destroy new cancer cells that develop intermittently in your body. The best stages for your health are the deeper stages three and four, stages during which higher levels of growth hormone and interleukins are released.

REM sleep accounts for about 25 percent of a normal sleep period. You have probably heard of REM sleep. REM stands for "rapid eye movement." It is in this period that you do most of your dreaming. When someone is in REM sleep, you can see that person's eyes darting around beneath the eyelids. During REM sleep, the brain is active but most of the body is paralyzed. This paralysis prevents one from acting out dreams (although dreams do occur to a smaller degree in non-REM sleep as well).

In REM sleep, your brain consolidates and processes newly learned information. Recent experiences and thoughts are replayed over and over, allowing neural networks to form new paths and make tighter connections. This is an important feature of memory consolidation. If you don't get a good night's sleep, your memory of what you learned that day will probably not be retained for very long. REM is just as important for learning factual information as it is for learning and remembering muscle tasks such as playing a new song on the piano or perfecting a golf swing.

During REM sleep, your brain also solves problems. Many of you have probably had that Aha! experience—you know, the one when you wake up and discover that you suddenly have the solution to a problem that had you stumped the night before. That is the benefit of REM sleep. Your brain truly functions better with a good night's sleep. When you are confronted with a new situation and are not sure what to do about it, "sleep on it." This may well bring you closer to your answer.

A typical night's sleep consists of five or six cycles through non-REM and REM sleep every ninety minutes. In the first cycle, when you reach REM sleep, you will be in it for only about thirty seconds. However, each time you complete a cycle, you spend longer amounts of time in REM sleep until you get about thirty minutes of REM sleep toward the end of a typical eight-hour sleep period.

Conversely, the deeper non-REM stages of sleep (three and four) occur in the earlier half of your sleep. A young, healthy adult will generally spend 5 percent of his or her time in stage one, 50 percent in stage two, 20 percent in stages three and four, and 25 percent in REM sleep.

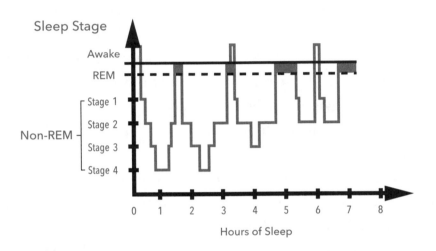

Clearly, sleep is important. The average American adult spends 7 to 7 ½ hours per night sleeping. In 1910, the average American adult slept 9 hours per night. This difference in sleep duration is thought to be related at least partly to the invention of the lightbulb. Interestingly, Thomas Edison had insomnia! The National Sleep Foundation published a survey a few years ago that found that 50 percent of American adults suffer from some form of insomnia at least a few times a week. The frequency of insomnia increases with age: two thirds of older adults struggle with some form of it. Fortunately, sleep is not entirely optional and your brain will force you to get at least some sleep whether you want to or not. How does your body do that? One major way your body is forced to sleep is through fluctuating its core body temperature. The hypothalamus, deep in the brain, causes body temperature to fluctuate by a degree and a half over a twenty-four-hour period.

Typically, your body temperature is at its lowest at around 4 A.M. If you are trying to stay up all night, this is when you are most likely to lose the battle. After this low point, the temperature starts to climb, you become more alert, and eventually you get up and start your day. Your body temperature peaks around 10 A.M., when you typically feel most alert. It then hits a low point at around 2 P.M., when everyone experiences a little sleepiness. Then it rises again in the early evening at around 6 P.M.

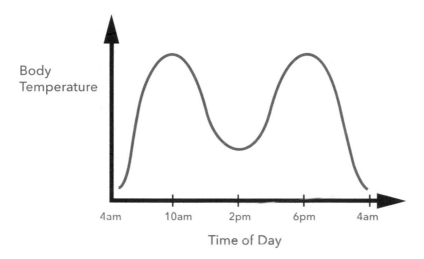

We all vary a little on exactly when we have peaks and valleys in our body temperature. This variation is what makes some people "night owls" and others "morning larks." An interesting recent discovery is that the hypothalamus is pretty much set in its pattern of body temperature fluctuations by the third month of a baby's life. In the various stages of life, there are also corresponding shifts in body temperature patterns. During adolescence, for example, the body temperature pattern shifts to the right and body temperature does not rise until later in the morning. This explains at least partially why your teenager doesn't want to get out of bed until noon. As people get older, the body temperature curve swings to the left; people tend to wake up earlier as they age.

The body temperature variations affect certain chemicals released in the brain stem that promote a sleepy state. The chemical adenosine makes you feel sleepy. Caffeine blocks adenosine receptors so your brain does not perceive as much adenosine, which is why it can keep you awake. Gamma-aminobutyric acid (GABA) makes you feel sleepy. Prescription sleeping pills target the GABA receptors, making it easier for the brain to perceive GABA, thereby inducing sleepiness.

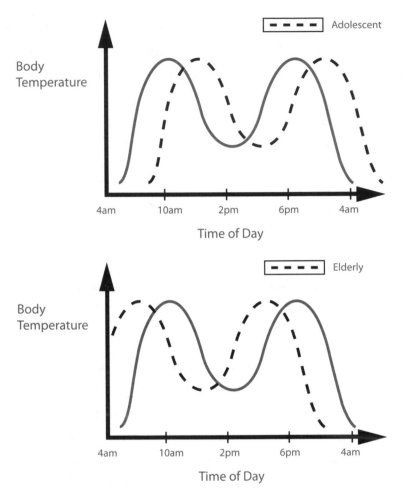

People's temperature fluctuations vary, as does their sensitivity to GABA and adenosine. People who have wide body temperature fluctuations are heavy sleepers, while those who have flatter body temperature fluctuations are lighter sleepers. With aging, body temperature fluctuations flatten. Exercise is the only known way to increase the fluctuations.

In addition to body temperature and brain chemicals such as GABA and adenosine, light has an effect on sleep physiology through a chemical called melatonin. Melatonin is made in the pineal gland of the brain, and it causes sleepiness. When your eyes are exposed to light, your pineal gland makes less melatonin, thus increasing your alertness.

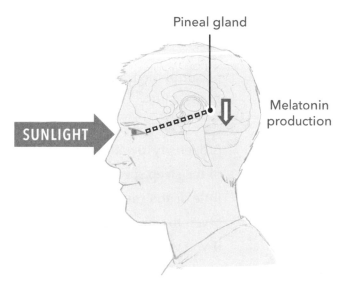

Melatonin production decreases with age; by age 60, you produce only 20 percent of your original level. This probably plays some role in why sleep is more difficult for the elderly.

So now you know what happens when you sleep. Is not getting enough sleep actually harmful to your health? The answer is yes. People do vary in how much they need to sleep in order to feel refreshed; however, a study done a few years ago at the Stanford Sleep Center determined that eight hours and fifteen minutes was the average amount of sleep required for the average person to stay awake in a darkened room in the middle of the afternoon without the aid of caffeine or other stimulants. If you start to dose off under these conditions, you are considered sleep-deprived.

Not getting enough sleep does have health consequences. Blood pressure rises, blood sugar rises, and the risk of having a heart attack increases. Remember all of the health consequences that accompany stress? They all happen with sleep deprivation, too. Why? Because a sleep deficit is interpreted by your body as stressful. Your cortisol levels rise, and your sympathetic nervous system fires. What's more, without a good night's sleep, you don't get the surge of growth hormone or the surge of immune-activating interleukins that you need. If that doesn't catch your interest, let me tell you about a study in 2008 that showed that

EEG Wave Patterns During Sleep

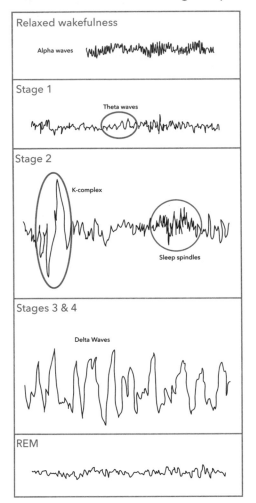

in rats subjected to sleep deprivation, newly born neurons sprouting in their little rat hippocampi died. Severe sleep deprivation can kill brain cells!

There are also studies that demonstrate a propensity toward weight gain on either extreme of the sleep spectrum. People who get either too little or too much sleep often put on weight, so seven to nine hours is a good target to shoot for if you want to avoid gaining weight.

Why would you gain weight if you are not sleeping enough? As I've mentioned before, research demonstrates a rise in several chemicals (such as cortisol, grehlin, galanin, and neuropeptide Y) when a person does not get enough sleep. These chemicals all stimulate the appetite and encourage overeating. If you are trying to lose weight, you are doing yourself a disservice if you do not get an adequate night's sleep on a regular basis.

Finally, more traffic accidents are caused by sleep deprivation than by alcohol intoxication. Sleep deprivation accounts for about 100,000 motor vehicle accidents per year in our country. Major national tragedies have been linked to sleep insufficiency, including the *Exxon Valdez* oil spill, the Chernobyl nuclear disaster, and the *Challenger* space shuttle tragedy.

Sleep Stages

RELAXED

When you are relaxed, your electroencephalogram (EEG) shows alpha-pattern brain waves. Your eyes are closed, but you are still awake.

NON-REM SLEEP

STAGE ONE

When you are in stage one, your EEG shows theta waves. Your body is relaxed, and you are drowsy; your body temperature drops. During this period, you are not officially sleeping. The average amount of time spent in this stage is 5 minutes.

STAGE TWO

This is considered the first stage of true sleep. Your EEG shows sleep spindles and K-complexes. Your heart rate and breathing slow down. The average time spent in this stage is 10 to 25 minutes initially, but you continue to cycle back to this stage intermittently throughout your sleep. If all you could achieve was stage two sleep, you would wake up feeling that you had slept, but you would not feel completely refreshed.

STAGES THREE AND FOUR

Your EEG shows an increase in delta waves, depending on whether you are in stage three or four. These are your deepest stages of sleep, when your heart rate, blood pressure, and respiratory rate are at their lowest. If you are not able to get enough of these stages of sleep one night, you body will spend more time in these deeper stages the next time you fall asleep in order to catch up.

REM SLEEP

During rapid eye movement (REM) sleep, your brain is very active, often dreaming, but your body is nearly paralyzed. Although the amount of time a person spends in the deeper non-REM stages of sleep decreases with age, the time an adult spends in REM sleep is fairly constant at about 20 to 25 percent throughout life. Actually, newborns spend 50 percent of their sleep time in REM sleep, but the amount drops to 20 to 25 percent by young adulthood. During REM sleep, your body temperature, heart rate, blood pressure, and respiratory rate all increase. It is in this phase that "nocturnal erections" (both penile and clitoral) occur. Generally, the brain passes through REM sleep three to five times a night, about every ninety minutes. At first the amount of time in REM is only a few minutes, but it increases with every cycle until the duration is about 30 minutes.

How Sleep Changes with Age

Newborns sleep eighteen hours a day and spend 50 percent of their sleeping time in REM sleep, consolidating the new information to which they have been exposed. Adults spend only 20 to 25 percent of their sleep time in REM sleep.

Children have extremely high melatonin levels at night. They pass really quickly into stages three and four sleep. Have you ever tried to wake a sleeping child? Children go right into deep sleep in no time!

Adolescents need one hour more of sleep than they did as children. As I've mentioned before, body temperature curves shift to the right in adolescence; some high schools now recognize this phenomenon and are starting classes later in the morning, when adolescents are more alert.

Young adults (ages 20 to 40). In your twenties and thirties you begin to lose the ability to descend into the deeply restorative stages three and four sleep. By age 40, stage four non-REM sleep has disappeared altogether. For women, hormonal fluctuations right before the menstrual cycle can also disrupt these sleep stages.

Midlife (ages 40 to 60). The midlife years show a further decline in the time spent in stage three sleep, and there are more nighttime awakenings. Body temperature variation starts to flatten in this stage of life, producing more shallow sleep. Exercise is always a great way to promote deeper sleep at any age, but in midlife and the later years, it can be especially helpful. Exercise increases the magnitude of daily body temperature fluctuation, so it helps people sleep more deeply. Those who are physically fit have deeper, more restorative sleep and fewer nighttime awakenings. Exercise is the only way adults can increase the amount of time spent in the deeper stages of sleep; fortunately, this benefit continues into the later years as well.

Later (age 60 and beyond). Men and women continue to spend 20 percent of their sleep in REM into the later years, but only 5 percent of non-REM sleep is spent in stage three. Also, as previously mentioned, the ability to enter stage four disappears by age forty. The body temperature curve typically shifts to the left at this time of life, so it is more common for older people to fall asleep sooner in the evening and awaken earlier in the morning. Advanced sleep stage syndrome occurs in 25 percent of people in this age group and causes very early morning awakening. Despite popular belief, people need the same amount of sleep when they're older as when they're younger. Many older people find it helpful to take short naps to catch up on their sleep.

The Epworth Sleepiness Scale

How likely are you to doze off or fall asleep in the following situations, in contrast to just feeling tired? Use the following scale to choose the most appropriate score for each situation:

0 = No chance of dozing

1 = Slight chance of dozing

2 = Moderate chance of dozing

3 = High chance of dozing

SITUATION	CHANCE OF DOZING
Sitting and reading	
Watching TV	
Sitting inactive in a public place (example: at a theater or in a meeting)	
As a passenger in a car for an hour without a break	
Lying down to rest in the afternoon when circumstances permit	
Sitting and talking to someone	
Sitting quietly after a lunch without alcohol	
In a car, while stopped for a few minutes in traffic	

1–6: Congratulations, you are getting enough sleep!

7–8: Your score is average.

9 and up: Seek the advice of a sleep specialist without delay.

HEALTHY SLEEP GUIDELINES

- **Get regular daily exercise.** This is one of the best ways to ensure healthy, good-quality sleep. As discussed, when you exercise, your body temperature fluctuations throughout the day become more accentuated. This allows your body to achieve the deeper stages three and four sleep, which are more rejuvenating for your body. In fact, exercise is the *only* known way to achieve longer and more frequent periods of stages three and four sleep.

- **Stick to a schedule** where you go to bed and get up at the same time every day. Going to bed at the same time every night is not as important as getting up at the same time every day, so if you want to get more sleep, it's better to go to bed earlier than to sleep in.

- **Avoid alcohol at night.** Alcohol is sedating; it induces stage two sleep, but it disrupts the deeper stages three and four. It is also metabolized quickly over a one- to two-hour period and, once metabolized, causes the release of a pulse of epinephrine that is stimulating and often wakes you up. Avoid alcohol at night this week and see if you sleep better.

- **Try to limit caffeine to no more than two cups of coffee before noon.** Caffeine is metabolized slowly, with a half-life of up to seven to twelve hours. This means that if you have four cups of coffee in the morning, you may still have the equivalent of two cups of coffee in your system when you go to bed at night.

- **Have a bedtime ritual.** Avoid paying bills or checking e-mail right before you go to bed. Stimulating mental activities right before bedtime make it harder for the brain to slow down and shift into sleep mood. Consider a warm bath as part of your bedtime ritual.

- **Reserve your bed for sleep and sex.** Don't use your bed to engage in mentally stimulating activities. You want your brain to associate your bed with relaxation and sleep.

- **Keep your bedroom environment optimal for sleeping.** Keep it uncluttered and without obvious work reminders. Your room should be dark, quiet, and on the cool side when you sleep. Consider trying earplugs, white noise, or eyeshades if you are sensitive to noise or light.

- If you find it hard to relax once you have gone to bed, **try slow, deep breathing.** Visualize a scene you find relaxing. You can also **try progressive muscle relaxation.** With this technique, you tighten up one area of the body such as your feet, concentrate on the tightness, then relax and concentrate on the heaviness of that part of the body. Work your way from one part of the body to the other. This is quite an old technique but works well for a lot of people.

- **Get rid of night worries.** If you tend to wake up in the middle of the night with racing thoughts or worries, keep paper and a pen by your bedside. Without even turning the light on, you can jot down the thought that woke you up. Tell yourself that you are going to let it go until the morning. This simple technique works amazingly well. It allows your brain to let go of the thought instead of dwelling on it.

- **Don't smoke.** Nicotine is a stimulant. Smokers who stop smoking notice that they sleep better.

- **Check your medications.** Over-the-counter medications such as decongestants can be stimulating, as can some prescription medications. If you have trouble sleeping, talk to your doctor about whether you should take your medication in the morning or evening.

- **Get out in the sun.** Sunlight naturally decreases your level of melatonin and increases alertness. Sunlight can help reprogram your brain's release of melatonin so that it occurs at night, when you want to sleep. If you are traveling eastward, expose yourself to afternoon sun to reset your biological clock. If you are traveling westward, expose yourself to morning sun.

- **Get up.** If you wake up in the middle of the night, don't lie there fretting about the time. Don't watch the clock; keep it turned around so you don't stare at it in desperation. If you can't fall asleep after about fifteen minutes (you don't know exactly because you aren't watching the clock, remember?), get up and leave your bed. Do something quietly until you feel drowsy. Most people choose to read quietly, but I would recommend that you use dim lighting if you do. Then get back into bed and see if you can fall asleep. What you don't want to do is to spend endless hours in bed agitating over how tired you are going to be the next day. As I said before, you want your brain to think of your bed as a place for relaxation and sleep, not to identify it as a torture chamber.

- **Avoid naps.** This is particularly important if you are trying to adjust to a particular sleep schedule at night.

- **Manage pain.** If pain frequently wakes you up at night, take an anti-inflammatory or acetaminophen before going to bed.

- **Limit fluids and diuretics in the evening** if frequent urination wakes you up.

- **Do not eat for three hours or drink fluids for two hours before lying down.** This will help you avoid problems with esophageal reflux. This goes for water too.

■ **Seek professional assistance.** If you are feeling overwhelmed by depression or anxiety, consider getting counseling and ask your doctor whether medication might be useful.

In really extreme cases of insomnia, an individual may be instructed to go to bed at 3 or 4 A.M. and to wake up at 6 A.M. Then, each subsequent night, the person is instructed to go to bed fifteen to thirty minutes earlier until a regular schedule is established. It sounds extreme, but it can sometimes work when nothing else does.

At times of high stress, also remember that even an ordinarily good sleeper may experience transient insomnia. Try not to focus too much on it, because your body will naturally front-load the deeper stages and REM sleep the next time you sleep. Transient insomnia usually doesn't last more than a few days to a few weeks, so your chances of getting back into a good sleeping pattern if you stick to a schedule are good. Try not to resort to caffeine in the morning or alcohol at night. Also, as hard as it might seem when you are tired, do try to stick with your daily exercise routine.

It's important for you to understand the connection between sleep and all the other aspects of your health. If you shortchange yourself on sleep, you shortchange yourself on all sorts of other important health matters as well.

Pablo, a 47-year-old ad salesman, traveled all the time, so his sleep cycle was a real problem. He found that when he traveled, he did best if he set his watch to the new time and refused to allow his mind to keep wandering back to what time it was back home. Also, once he arrived in his new location, he made sure he exposed himself to some sunlight (if there was any), and he never let himself take a nap. If he was exhausted, he went to bed early, but not before 8 P.M. local time. That way, he would be able to sleep through the night and adjust more quickly to the new time zone. He also tried to exercise every day even when he was traveling all over the world. This regimen really worked for him. He learned to adjust his internal clock to new time zones better than almost anyone else I have met.

NUTRITION: PROTEIN PEARLS

We've talked about two of the major macronutrients, fats and carbohydrates. Now let's take a look at the third one, protein. Protein is an essential nutrient. We can't live without it. Your body depends on protein for many important roles.

Proteins are constantly broken down in your body. In most instances, the proteins are retained and reused, but a continual supply of protein must be available to the body to replace what is lost. This process is referred to as protein turnover, and it takes place throughout your life. Without the proper amount of protein, growth and bodily functions would not be possible.

Most Americans get more than enough protein. The daily dietary requirement for an adult is .8 gram of protein per kilogram (2.2 pounds) of body weight. That equates to about 64 grams a day of protein for a 175-pound man and 47 grams a day for a 130-pound woman. Roughly, you can take your weight in pounds and divide that number in half, and that would be the number of grams of protein required in your diet. That's really not very much protein, and many Americans get double this amount. For example, a one-pound steak, not unusual in restaurants, supplies 100 grams of protein all by itself.

What foods contain protein? A three-ounce serving of meat, poultry, or fish will give you 21 grams of protein. Two eggs supply 14 grams; a cup of nonfat milk or yogurt, 8 grams. An ounce of cheese gives you 7 grams of protein, but remember, it also has a lot of saturated fat. An ounce of nuts gives you an average of 5 grams of protein. Nuts also contain a fair amount of fat; it is the good, unsaturated type, but it still provides a lot of calories, so you need to be careful with the portions. Beans give you about 9 grams of protein in a typical half-cup serving. There are also small amounts of protein in bread, pasta, and rice (3 grams in a typical slice or half-cup serving) as well as vegetables (2 grams in a cup [raw] or half-cup [cooked] serving.)

What exactly is a protein? The basic structural unit of protein is the amino acid. To form proteins, amino acids are combined into long chains. There are twenty different amino acids in all. Nine of them are essential, which means that the body cannot manufacture them. Therefore *they must come from food sources.* The eleven nonessential amino acids can be made by our bodies, *if* all the building blocks they need are available.

Animal sources of protein such as meat, poultry, fish, eggs, and dairy products provide all nine essential amino acids. For that reason they are often referred to as complete proteins. Virtually all proteins from animal sources are complete proteins. Plant proteins usually lack one or more of the essential amino acids and so are referred to as incomplete proteins. Soy, which provides all nine essential amino acids, is the exception. It is therefore important to have the right mix of plant proteins in your diet so that you can get the appropriate amounts of essential and nonessential amino acids.

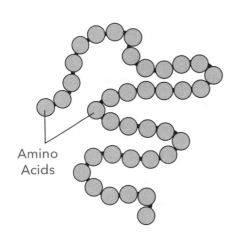

Amino Acids

Protein Molecule

Vegetarians can receive adequate protein if their food sources are varied and their caloric needs are met. Also, vegetarians often eat eggs and dairy products, which contain complete protein. In truth, a vegetarian diet is healthier than an animal-based diet because the animal sources of protein all contain saturated fat, which, as you know by now, is not considered healthful. The exception to the rule is the egg, which has more saturated than saturated fat; it is high in cholesterol, though, with 200 milligrams of cholesterol in each egg (300 milligrams being the daily total recommended amount). Remember, though, that cholesterol is affected more by the saturated and trans fats in your diet than by the amount of cholesterol. Remember, too, that fish does not have much saturated fat; it has mainly healthy unsaturated fat. If you want to continue to keep animal products in your diet but you do not want to sacrifice health, eat nonfat dairy products, go light on cheese, take the skin off turkey and chicken, and avoid red meat or eat it sparingly. The leanest grades of meat are "select" and "choice." The leanest cuts are loin, flank, and round.

Many people wonder if they need more protein when they increase the amount of exercise they do. Most Americans get more than enough protein for even the most vigorous exercise. Endurance athletes may need more protein, but their higher caloric intake generally supplies it. The normal protein requirements are met if 11 percent of the calories on a maintenance diet come from protein. In the average American diet 15 percent of calories come from protein. Nevertheless, many athletes, hoping to build muscle, consume high-protein powders, drinks, and bars. It is important to know that protein by itself will not build muscle unless you work out. When you eat more protein than you need, it's broken down and the excess calories are stored as body fat, not as a reserve supply of protein. Your Personal Nutrition Plan is calculated to deliver 25 percent of your calories from protein, so if you are following this plan, you shouldn't need to add extra protein. Just know that when you eat too many calories from anything, whether it is protein, carbohydrates, or fat, the excess calories that are not burned for energy will be stored as fat.

The good thing about protein is that it is filling and creates a slow, gradual rise in blood sugar. When you eat protein, your stomach empties more slowly, so it leaves you feeling full longer. Perhaps for this reason, high-protein diets have recently been found to be the diets most associated with long-term weight loss. The important thing to note, though, is that true weight loss (that is, body fat loss) is still going to depend upon your achieving a calorie deficit. You will be less likely to achieve this if you consume high-fat protein sources because every gram of fat has so many more calories than carbohydrates or protein. The best diet for your heart and for your overall health is one in which protein is derived mainly from plant sources or fish, thereby lowering saturated fats and increasing unsaturated fats.

TIPS FOR CHOOSING HEALTHY PROTEIN

HEALTHY RECOMMENDATIONS

- Choose fish, shellfish, and skinless poultry. White poultry meat has less fat than dark meat.

- When having beef, pick lean meats and remove visible fat. Focus on lean beef such as round, sirloin, chuck, and loin. Buy choice or select grades of beef rather than prime. Lean beef should be more than 85 percent lean.

- Try to eat two servings of baked or grilled oily fish each week. Choose fish high in omega-3 fatty acids, such as mackerel, lake trout, herring, sardines, albacore tuna, anchovies, and salmon.

- Add low-sodium, low-fat seasonings to food such as spices, herbs, and other flavorings when cooking or eating.

- Consume meat substitutes such as beans, lentils, or tofu in entrées, salads, or soups.

- Choose lean veal, ham, pork, or lamb.

- Pick sandwich meats that are lower in fat, such as turkey, chicken, turkey ham, turkey pastrami, and ham.

- Try meat alternatives such as tofu, tempeh, soy hot dogs, and soy burgers.

PORTION SIZES AND PREPARATION TIPS

- A three-ounce portion of cooked meat is about the size of a deck of cards or the palm of your hand.

- Beans, eggs, nuts, seeds, peanut butter, and tofu are all great meat alternatives that are rich in protein.

- Prepare meats by grilling, baking, broiling, roasting, poaching, microwaving, or stir-frying. Avoid adding sauces, creams, or gravies and frying foods.

- When roasting a whole chicken or turkey, you can cook it with the skin on to retain moisture; then remove the skin before serving the meat. Choose poultry that has not been injected with fats or broths.

- Increase the volume of omelets by using only one egg yolk and adding extra egg whites. Eat egg yolks in moderation, especially if you have an elevated cholesterol level.

This week, pay attention to what kinds of proteins are in your diet. Experiment with ways of eating more protein with unsaturated fat and less protein with saturated fat.

FITNESS: FLEXIBILITY EXERCISES

Staying flexible is important so that your joints can move freely. When your joint motion is full, your entire body can move more efficiently.

When doing stretches, it is important to remember that they should never be painful. You should always feel a "gentle stretch." Ideally, stretching should be performed when there is increased blood flow through the muscles—for example, at the end of a workout. However, if you stretch gently and regularly, you can stretch anytime safely. When you are stretching, it is best to hold each stretch for at least 30 seconds and repeat each stretch two times. One more tip: Even though you are holding one position for an extended period of time, don't hold your breath. Breathe deeply and regularly to enhance the relaxation and stretch.

Quadriceps Stretch

The first stretch is the Quadriceps Stretch. The quadriceps is the big muscle in the front of your thigh. This muscle can become tight if you sit a lot during the day, so for most people it's a good muscle to stretch. This stretch will have you standing on one foot at a time, so if you need help with balance, you might like to have a desk or wall nearby. Stand with a chair right behind you. Place the top of your right foot on the chair, or grasp your right ankle with your right hand. Tighten your abdomen and buttocks, and point your bent knee directly toward the ground. You should feel a stretch in the front of your thigh. Repeat on the other side.

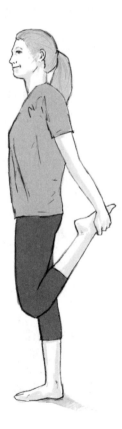

STANDING HAMSTRING STRETCH

Now we will move to the opposite side of your thigh and focus on the hamstring. This muscle can be stretched a number of different ways, but since you are already standing, we will review the Standing Hamstring Stretch. Turn around so you are facing the chair. Place one heel on the chair. If the chair is too high, you can use anything lower—a step stool, for example. With your foot up, keep your hips square, your chest lifted, and your knee as straight as possible. Ideally, the knee of the leg you are standing on should be slightly flexed. In this position, most people will feel the stretch behind the knee and thigh. If you do not feel a stretch in this position, you may need to lean your chest slightly forward until you can feel the stretch. Repeat on the other side. The hamstring is an important muscle to stretch because it can limit the movement of your hip if it is tight. If your hip can't move through a full range of motion, your lower back must compensate for it—and we all know how prevalent lower-back pain is today.

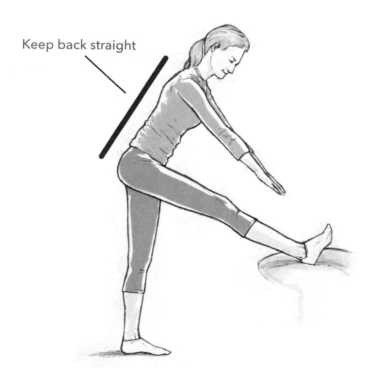

Keep back straight

CALF STRETCH

Next we'll move on to the lower leg with the Calf Stretch. This muscle group is responsible for supporting us with standing and walking, and therefore it is used throughout the day, every day. It is also the most common place for a "charley horse" or cramping to occur. The best way to relieve and prevent such cramping is by stretching. Let's stick with the standing position and review how to stretch the calf in this position. Stand about two steps away from a wall or a chair, facing it. Place your feet in a "stride-step" position and place your hands on the wall or a chair. Keep your back heel on the ground as you bend your front knee until you feel a stretch in the lower part of the back leg. Be careful not to arch your lower back. Repeat on the other side.

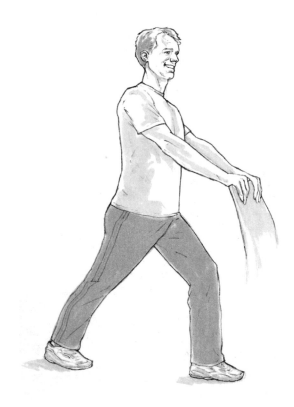

Doorway Chest Stretch

Let's work up from the lower body and stretch the chest. This is the last of our standing stretches. Stand in the doorway of a room. Place your forearms up against each jamb with your elbows just below shoulder height. Step one foot forward and slowly transfer your weight onto your front foot until you feel a stretch in your chest and the front of your shoulders. This Doorway Chest Stretch is important for anyone who spends a lot of time sitting at a desk or driving a car. This position encourages the spine to flex forward and the back muscles to over-stretch, while the muscles in the front shorten. Over time, these muscles adapt to this position and become weak and painful. Stretching the chest muscles is one way to counteract this and improve your posture.

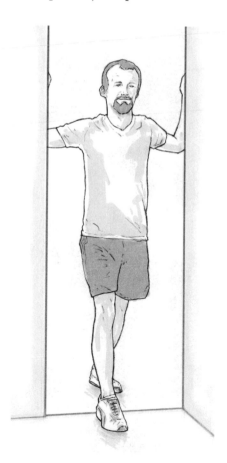

PIRIFORMIS (GLUTEAL) STRETCH

Now let's move on to some stretches you can do while sitting in a chair. Ideally, the chair you use should be a firm, supportive one. The first stretch is the Piriformis (Gluteal) Stretch. Sit on the edge of a chair. Cross your right leg over the left and place your right ankle on your left knee. Sit up tall and gently press your right knee toward the chair until you feel a stretch in the outer part of your right hip. If you don't feel a stretch with this method, try this: sit up straight and pull your right knee toward your left shoulder until you feel a stretch in the right gluteal region. Repeat on the other side. The piriformis is a muscle on top of the sciatic nerve. If this muscle is tight, it can possibly bind down onto the sciatic nerve, creating symptoms of sciatica, or pain, numbness, and/or tingling, down into the leg. Stretching is a great way to prevent or relieve this.

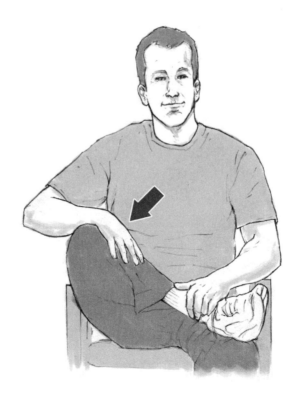

Upper Trapezius (Neck) Stretch

For most people, the neck and upper-back muscles create feelings of pain and tightness. We will review two stretches to address these problem areas. The first is the Upper Trapezius (Neck) Stretch. This muscle runs from the top of your neck down into the top of your shoulders. Sit on the edge of a chair with both feet flat on the ground. Slowly tip your left ear toward your left shoulder. Keeping your shoulders relaxed, reach over the top of your head and place the palm of your left hand on the right side of your head. Gently add a bit more pressure with your hand until you feel a stretch on the side of your neck. It is important not to use too much pressure or overstretch this area, so be very gentle! Repeat on the other side.

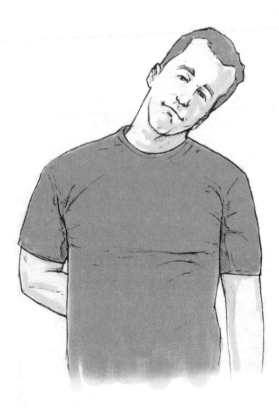

LEVATOR SCAPULAE STRETCH

The levator scapulae is a muscle that runs from the back of your skull to the upper corner of your shoulder blade. When tight, it can cause neck pain, headache, and sometimes a "knot" in the corner of the shoulder blade. To stretch this muscle, you start the same way as the last stretch. Sit up tall, and instead of bringing your ear to your shoulder, turn your head and direct your nose toward your left elbow with your arms resting at your sides. Then place the palm of your left hand on the right side of the back of your head. Apply gentle pressure until you feel a stretch anywhere from your neck down into the top of your right shoulder blade. Remember to be very gentle with your pressure! Repeat on the other side.

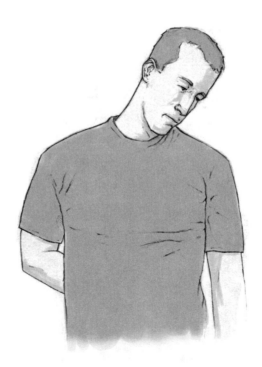

Latissimus Dorsi Stretch

The last stretch we will review is for a muscle group not really known for its pain or tightness. However, if the latissimus dorsi muscle in your middle and lower back becomes tight, your shoulder and spine motion can be limited and therefore dysfunctional. Most people find this stretch particularly relaxing, so it is a nice stretch to perform throughout a workday. Sit on the edge of a chair with your feet flat on the ground. Place your right hand on your upper thigh. Raise your left hand over your head. Keeping your abdominals in, reach your left hand up to the ceiling and then over to the right side, feeling a stretch on your left side. Breathe deeply while you hold this stretch. Repeat on the other side.

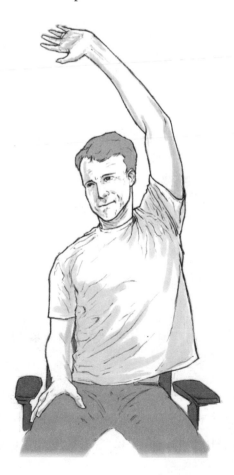

You have now practiced eight stretches that you can do anywhere—at work, at home, or on the go. If you don't want to do them all at once, try breaking them up. You can spread them out during the day. For example, you can perform the standing stretches at home after your shower and the sitting stretches at work after lunch. This way, you get the benefits of stretching without having to take much time to fit it in. The most important thing is to find the best way to make it work for you.

FLEXIBILITY EXERCISES: A QUICK REVIEW

Quadriceps Stretch

Standing Hamstring Stretch

Calf Stretch

Doorway Chest Stretch

Piriformis (Gluteal) Stretch

Upper Trapezius (Neck) Stretch

Levator Scapulae Stretch

Latissimus Dorsi Stretch

LEARN IT!

- Non-REM sleep (stages one, two, three, and four) makes up 75 percent of a normal sleep period.

- Growth hormone and interleukins are released during stages three and four sleep. These chemicals repair the wear and tear damage and help the immune system stay strong.

- Rapid eye movement (REM) sleep accounts for 25 percent of a normal sleep period.

- REM sleep is important for memory and problem solving.

- You need seven to nine hours of sleep every night.

- If you don't get enough sleep, you run the risk of weight gain, increased blood sugar, increased blood pressure, and increased likelihood of heart attacks and depression.

- Adults require .8 gram of protein per kilogram (2.2 pounds) of body weight; for example, 64 grams daily for a 175-pound man, 47 grams daily for a 130-pound woman.

- When you eat more protein than you need, it is broken down and stored as body fat, not as a reserve supply of protein.

- Protein is made up of amino acids. Nine amino acids are essential, meaning the body cannot make them and they must come from food. Eleven amino acids are nonessential; they can be made by the body.

- Animal protein is a complete protein because it contains all of the nine essential amino acids.

- Plant protein is usually incomplete because it lacks one or more of the essential amino acids. If you do not eat any animal products, you must eat a variety of plant foods to make sure you get all of the essential amino acids in your diet.

PERSONALIZE IT!

This week, work on your Learning Brain.

Your brain has a tremendous capacity to learn. Enhance factors that optimize learning. That is, get adequate sleep, minimize stress, and exercise regularly. Remember to repeat over and over whatever it is you want your brain to memorize. Your brain is also playful. It loves puzzles, humor, and questions. Finally, don't be afraid to make mistakes. Your brain learns from them, so they are an important part of growing.

Here are some examples of how people in The Program have personalized this brain principle and put it into action.

- John C., a 63-year-old business executive, took forty-five-minute power naps in the afternoon to recharge his battery and keep his brain in high gear. Sleeping helped him be more creative in problem solving both at work and at home.

- Carrie B., a 29-year-old mother of one, found that she could learn best from mistakes and mishaps if she wrote them down in her "challenges and opportunities" journal, where she could record things that did not go as planned and how she might do things differently in the future if a similar situation presented itself. She also wrote down one positive thing she learned from each mistake.

- Angie M., a 44-year-old graphic designer, found that for her the key to learning was mastering stress. If she was anxious, she could not learn. If she was relaxed, she could concentrate and learn much better. Angie learned how to destress in seconds by taking slow, deep breaths and then picturing her family in their backyard playing with their golden retriever. When she pictured this, she could calm herself from the often inconsequential thing she was stressing over. Once she calmed down, she could think more clearly and rationally, allowing for better coping skills and problem solving.

LIVE IT!

- Review last week's goals and create this week's short-term goals.

- Focus on sleep this week. If sleep is an issue for you, decide which sleeping tips you would like to try.

- Identify where you get the majority of your protein. Is it mainly from animals or plants? How much fat does it contain, and is it saturated or unsaturated fat?

- Decide when you would like to do a few minutes of gentle stretching each day and begin to incorporate flexibility exercises into your routine. You can stretch at home or at work, all at once or intermittently throughout the day.

HAPPINESS AND YOUR HEALTH

Nothing happens until something moves.

—ALBERT EINSTEIN

DON'T WORRY, BE HAPPY! It sounds so simple, but feeling happy isn't always so easy. This week we're going to take a look at mood disorders such as depression and anxiety, conditions that affect so many Americans. The fact is that 18 percent of the U.S. population suffers from anxiety every year and 17 percent of Americans will experience major depression at some point in their lifetime. In this chapter, I'm going to show you how depression is influenced by chemicals in your brain, but, more important, I'm going to show you how you can significantly influence these chemicals through your lifestyle. Your mood has as much physiology behind it as anything else in your body, and it's an important piece of your overall health.

Let's begin by putting one myth to rest. Mood disorders such as depression and anxiety are not conditions you should just tough out. They are real, physiologic conditions with physiologic consequences. We now know that the longer it takes a person suffering from a major depression to get into remission, the more diffi-cult it is to get that person into remission. Did you know that the longer a person spends in a major depressive episode, the more likely it is that he or she will suffer a recurrent episode? What's more, future depressive episodes can be triggered by stressors that ordinarily wouldn't have led to such a major depressive reaction. So if you have had persistently sad feelings for more than a couple of weeks, particularly if they are associated with feelings of hopelessness, worthlessness, and appetite or sleep changes, and obviously if you have had suicidal thoughts, you should not hesitate to speak to your doctor. Depression is not uncommon, and it is treatable with both medication and nonmedication therapies. The sooner you recover, the better your long-term prognosis.

Think back to Week 3, when we reviewed the overall structure of the brain. There are the reptilian brain stem, the mammalian limbic system, and the highly developed outer brain, the cerebral cortex. The limbic system and the cerebral cortex are tightly interconnected, and both play a role in depression and anxiety and in the successful treatment of these conditions.

The limbic system in the core of your brain houses a lot of mood-active structures. The amygdala, in the limbic system, is the center for emotionally charged memories and persistent negative thoughts. It is active during stress, anxiety, and depression. It sits conveniently beside the hippocampus, the part of the brain that serves long-term memory. The hippocampus is tightly connected to the hypothalamus, an important area in all sorts of body regulations. When you are stressed, anxious, or depressed, the hypothalamus tells the pituitary to tell the adrenal gland to produce cortisol. This hypothalamus-pituitary-adrenal (HPA) axis is therefore the highway for the stress response as well as for depression and anxiety. Chronic activation of the adrenal gland, as you may recall from the lesson on stress, has wide ramifications on your body's health. So *with depression, just as with stress, there is an increased risk of diabetes, hypertension, heart attacks, strokes, immune dysfunction, and obesity.*

Mood and Gender

Depression and anxiety affect twice as many women as men.

Manic-depressive disorder is strongly linked to genes and affects men and women equally.

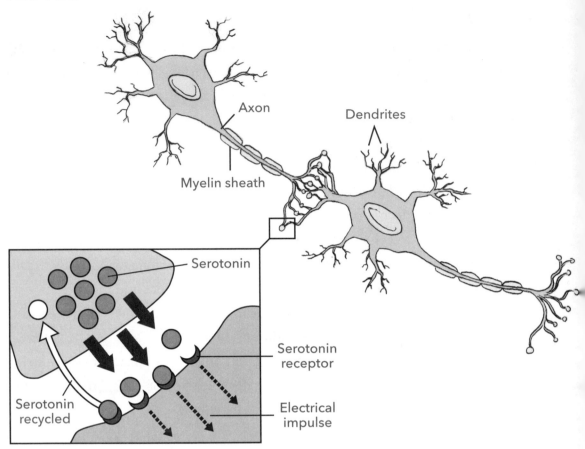

Now let's talk about mood chemicals in the brain. The chemicals I am referring to are neurotransmitters, which are released from one neuron to the next.
Neurotransmitters are messengers that tell the nerve cell next in line what to do.
They tell the nerve whether it should or shouldn't pass a message along. They also
influence the production of other chemicals inside the neuron.

The major neurotransmitters in the brain are glutamate, an excitatory neurotransmitter, and gamma-aminobutyric acid (GABA), an inhibitory neurotransmitter. There is a fine balance between the two. Glutamate is essential for learning,
but if the level becomes too high, it injures and even kills neurons. For example,
toxic glutamate levels cause much of the damage in a stroke. First, neurons die
because the artery that normally brings in nutrients suddenly shuts down from a
clot. When these cells die, they release their stockpile of glutamate, which kills all

the surrounding neurons. GABA is important too. When people have a low GABA level, they feel anxious. Benzodiazepine medications such as Valium, Ativan, and Xanax, which are sometimes prescribed for anxiety, stimulate the GABA receptors. The relaxation you feel after you have had a good workout occurs in part because your GABA levels increase when you exercise.

You can see how important it is to maintain the right balance between glutamate and GABA. You should know, however, that although these two neurotransmitters are the most plentiful in your brain, they are really considered to be the work crew in this story. There are three other neurotransmitters—serotonin, dopamine, and norepinephrine—that really run the show. Although only 1 percent of the brain is devoted to producing these chemicals, they determine the balance of glutamate and GABA levels and therefore influence your mood. Serotonin is calming and mood-elevating. Norepinephrine drives alertness and energy. Dopamine promotes motivation, attention, and pleasure.

In depression, serotonin, norepinephrine, and dopamine levels drop and the glutamate level rises. Perhaps more important, the level of brain-derived neurotrophic factor (BDNF) drops. This chemical is critical to cell survival, and when the BDNF level decreases, the nerve cells start to atrophy and die. When the BDNF level increases, the nerve cells thrive and grow, branching out nerve fibers that connect with other surrounding nerve fibers. BDNF also promotes the production of new neurons, something that we have only recently discovered. In depression, chronic stress, and chronic pain, the BDNF level drops, and, what is most stunning of all, imaging studies show that when this happens for long enough the hippocampus and frontal cortex in the brain can actually shrink in size!

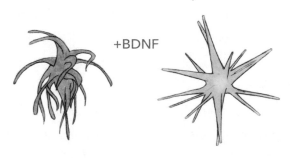

+BDNF

The good news in all this is that there are some very concrete things you can do to reverse this process. Antidepressant medications raise serotonin, norepinephrine, dopamine, and BDNF levels. With higher levels of BDNF, hippocampal cells start to regenerate. Reduction of glutamate and cortisol levels (as seen in the successful treatment of depression) also allows for a return to normal BDNF levels. With successful treatment, there is not only an improvement in mood but also a reduction in the physical consequences of depression as well. Specifically, pain often decreases with a return to normal levels of serotonin.

What else can both increase brain-derived growth factor and improve hippocampal recovery? Exercise. Just like antidepressants, exercise raises serotonin, norepinephrine, dopamine, and BDNF levels. Exercise has a tremendous influence on your brain chemicals and your mood. In fact, a 1999 study at Duke University showed that exercise was better than Zoloft, an antidepressant, in lifting mood and treating depression in the long term. I certainly think there are times when medication is appropriate for treating mood—not only appropriate but very beneficial—but I think it is remarkable how little attention is given to exercise and how extraordinary it is in reshaping the brain. Part of the reason you hear more about medications than exercise is that there is not the same kind of marketing money spent on exercise as there is on drug promotion. You can exercise for free. Also, people tend to look for the easier way out when it comes to most things, and it is certainly easier to swallow a pill than go out for a run.

You don't, however, get all of the benefits from a pill that you would get if you took the extra time and energy to exercise. If you do take medication for your mood, exercise will make things that much better. It will help lift your mood, raise your level of neurotransmitters, boost your BDNF level, stimulate brain growth, and speed remission while preventing future relapses. The BDNF increase from exercise will help you increase the areas of higher thinking in your frontal cortex so that you can better control aberrant moods and thoughts. But even if a person makes more BDNF through exercise or medications, you still need to tell your brain where to lay down new nerve networks. This is where counseling comes in.

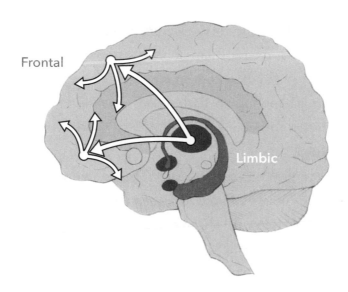

Frontal

Limbic

Learning why you do what you do and how you might respond differently can make all the difference when it comes to treating depression or anxiety. Combined with BDNF, new ways of thinking can create new pathways to serve as alternate routes for processing information and influencing what happens in the limbic system.

Remember, the limbic system reaches out and connects to the cerebral cortex. They talk to each other. You can experience the same situation one day and see it as gloomy, yet on another day see it in a much sunnier light. That change in perception is due to the changing conversations between your limbic system and cerebral cortex. You can influence your mood by changing your cerebral cortex's input or by altering your limbic system's activity (through the techniques we discussed in Week 3 under stress management).

A condition you hear a lot about is attention deficit disorder (ADD) or attention-deficit-hyperactivity disorder (ADHD). In this condition, the dopamine level is low. Your dopamine level controls your motivation. You need to have a high enough amount of dopamine to hold your attention. Some people create all kinds of stressors in their lives or turn to risk-taking behaviors to deal with chronically low dopamine levels. Others stall before deadlines because they have learned that last-minute stress helps them focus. Medication given for ADD/ADHD works by raising dopamine levels; exercise can do this, too. Dopamine, like most chemicals in your body, does best when kept in a certain range; not too high, not too low. Dopamine levels are too low in Parkinson's disease and too high in schizophrenia. You will hear more about dopamine next week, when we discuss the physiology of addiction.

Now that you understand the chemistry behind depression, you might ask why some people have problems with depression and others don't. Part of the reason is genetics. If you struggle with chronic depression, you may not produce sufficient serotonin or norepinephrine. Or you may have receptors that respond too much or too little to individual neurotransmitters.

Yet even with a very normal baseline production of neurotransmitters and normal receptor activity, chronic stressors or chronic pain can alter your brain's physiology, allowing major depression to develop. In other words, external events play a big role in your mood; it is certainly not all about genetics. For example, if your environment is too stressful for too long, the high levels of cortisol you produce may shrivel your hippocampus, and make it less able to regulate mood chemicals such as serotonin. This can happen to you as an adult. It can also happen to an unborn child if the pregnant mother is subjected to extreme amounts of stress. If a pregnant rat is placed under a lot of stress, the mother rat's cortisol crosses the placenta and enters the unborn baby rat's brain, shrinking the unborn baby's hippocampus. These rat babies are born more anxious because their mood regulation system has been disrupted. Fortunately, if the babies are placed in a calm, supportive, nurturing environment after birth, their brains can be reshaped and the condition corrected.

There are also studies linking decreases in serotonin levels to rapidly falling estrogen levels in women's perimenopausal period, suggesting that sudden estrogen drops can contribute to mood issues. Finally, certain medications can cause mood changes, as can certain medical conditions, so if you are struggling with your mood, make sure you mention this to your doctor so he or she can help you sort things out.

Anxiety

Anxiety is more common than you may realize. It affects 40 million Americans, or 18 percent of the population. Some people are born with physiology that makes it harder for them to feel calm; for example, some people are born with slightly altered GABA receptors so the calming, Valium-like chemical (which everyone's brain naturally produces) does not bind very well. Other times, traumatic events in a person's life cause the amygdala to develop a quick trigger, and even a small amount of stress stimulates a big stress response.

Regardless of the cause, know that there are several very effective treatments for anxiety. One of the most effective things you can do for anxiety is to do a lot of moderately intense physical exercise, which does a lot to boost the calming, feel-good chemicals in the brain. *Exercise actually promotes a physical restructuring of the brain.* Exercise helps neurons (that have shriveled due to stress chemicals) thrive and branch again, so when you exercise, it promotes brainpower not only to learn better but to develop better neural patterns for coping as well.

Counseling can also help. There are several methods counselors use to help people move past specific or even general situations that trigger anxiety. Finally, medication can help particularly if combined with both physical activity and counseling.

Chronic Pain

Chronic pain is a subject that deserves more attention than it gets. The brain and body are highly interconnected, and when people have chronic pain there is a lot of interplay in several areas of health. Chronic pain activates the brain's stress center. This can result in the depletion of certain neurotransmitters, causing depression or anxiety to develop. The depression, in turn, makes the pain feel even more intense. Pain may cause sleep disruption. The sleep disruption, in turn, can intensify the pain and worsen mood issues. Sleep is also important for repairing all the wear and tear that goes on in your body daily, as we saw in Week 7; it is necessary for keeping your immune system strong so it can fight off infections and even prevent cancer.

Treatment of chronic pain is therefore necessary not just for the relief of pain but to protect one's overall health as well. If you suffer from chronic pain, know that there are treatments available to help with the pain and also with mood issues or sleep disruption. These treatments may include medication, but exercise is a very potent therapy for pain as well. Stress management techniques such as meditation and yoga can be helpful, too. There are also medical centers that specialize in pain management; treatments include alternative therapies such as acupuncture, acupressure, or deep forms of massage. You don't need to suffer silently.

Here's more good news. There are hundreds of different studies that show that how you choose to live your life—what you do and how you decide to think—plays an enormous role in your ability to be happy. In other words, you are not just a victim of chemicals floating around in your head. You can take some very concrete steps to take the reins of your life and improve your mood. It is extremely important to remember that our lives are not wholly predetermined by our genes. For example, the environment you are exposed to influences whether certain genes are turned on or off. Your behaviors can also turn genes on or off. So can your thoughts. You can have much more influence over your mood than you may have thought.

Here are the top ten Happiness Strategies that have been scientifically documented to improve mood.

- **Count your blessings and appreciate what you have.** Every day, either write down three things you are grateful for or tell them to your partner or a close friend. People who actively focus on what is going right in their lives become happier people. The more you think this way, the more your brain will lay down new nerve paths and the more reflexive and second nature this positive way of thinking will become.

- **Practice optimism.** Expect positive outcomes. Always try to see the best in people, situations, and circumstances. You don't have to be a Pollyanna, nor should you be unrealistic, but there are always two sides—good and bad—to a person, situation, or circumstance. Focus on the good. Optimistic thoughts are often self-fulfilling. When people are optimistic and believe that something good will come of what they are working toward, they are more likely to persevere when they hit roadblocks. Their resilience and persistence are what lead them to succeed.

- **Focus on your own life and making it everything you want it to be.** Don't compare yourself to other people. Whenever you see yourself start to make comparisons, stop. Shift back to your own life. In the end, if you are happy and fulfilled with what you are doing, it doesn't matter what anybody else is doing. People who live life without making comparisons are happier.

- **Surround yourself with loving, supportive, positive friends and family.** Human beings have evolved to be part of a bigger network. Social interactions change the very chemistry within your body. In your brain, serotonin and dopamine levels increase in response to positive social interactions. In women, positive social interactions cause oxytocin levels to rise, and, in men, vasopressin levels rise. Oxytocin and vasopressin are the "tend and befriend" chemicals that drive people toward tighter social connections. People with strong, supportive social networks live healthier, happier, longer lives.

- **Learn to manage stress.** Stress plays a pivotal role in initiating depression because the high cortisol levels associated with stress disrupt the brain's ability to modulate the feel-good chemicals of serotonin, norepinephrine, and dopamine.

- **Live in the present.** Enjoy the moment. Stop thinking so much about everything you need to do tomorrow. Savor the little things along the way, like the way the grass smells when you leave for work in the morning or how comfortable it feels to sit down and relax at the end of a day. Don't be afraid to be frivolous, either. You don't have to be serious all the time. It's okay to watch a mindless sitcom and just laugh. Your brain loves to play. Let it.

- **Strive to be part of something bigger than yourself.** Work toward something in which you find significant meaning. People who turn their focus away from themselves and toward something in which they find true meaning often find themselves happier and more passionate about life in general. If you are looking for a job, look for a company that has a mission statement that involves a more meaningful pursuit than a purely financial one. Studies show that employees who feel their jobs are meaningful on a deeper level are happier.

- **Volunteer.** Helping others increases happiness. Become involved with something you feel deeply about, such as global poverty, health, education, the environment, or disadvantaged children. There are many areas in which you can make a difference. People are happier giving than receiving. In a study published in *Science* in 2008, investigators asked forty-six participants to rate their happiness in the morning, gave each of them some money, and then randomly assigned them to spend the money on themselves or on others. When participants rated their happiness at the end of the day, the amount of money they had received was unrelated to their happiness. Those who spent the money on themselves had no increase in happiness, but those who spent it on others had significantly higher happiness ratings. Buying things for yourself or receiving gifts may bring happiness briefly, but once you get past the basic essentials for survival, such as food, clothing, and shelter, material wealth does not translate into happiness. After an initial burst of pleasure, people quickly revert back to their baseline level of happiness. This also happens when someone loses money or material wealth. With loss, people are sad at first, but then they revert back to their baseline level of happiness.

- **Learn to accept what you can't change.** Try to let go of things over which you have no control. If you can accept that there are things in life that aren't always ideal but that life can be good anyway, you've taken a giant step closer to happiness.

- **Finally, work exercise into your daily routine.** I've saved this one for last because this is the most tangible of the ten strategies to improve your happiness. As discussed above, when you exercise, you change the chemistry in your brain, but, more important, you ultimately change the very structure of your brain.

In all of the strategies I've just mentioned, repetition is required so that there is strong and consistent signaling to stimulate the brain to strengthen the synapses of existing nerve connections and to build up new and improved networks.

So here's the question: Is happiness important to your health? Absolutely! Happy people are physically healthier. Happy people live longer. Happy people enjoy a higher quality of life. There's one thing for sure: *the brain and body are inextricably connected.* You can't address the body without addressing the brain, and vice versa. If you want to be happy and enjoy optimal health, you need to take care of both.

Feeling the Energy

It's important to surround yourself with positive people. Of course you want to be there for a friend who is going through a hard time, but did you know that another person's mood can affect the beat-to-beat variability in your heart? I find this extraordinary. Everybody has variations in their heart's beat-to-beat variability. That's normal. The pattern of that beat-to-beat variability can indicate whether if you are in a happy, healthy mood or not. Your brain and heart are both powered by electrical activity (that's what is being measured when you get an EEG or ECG). If you remember physics, you'll remember that electrical current generates electromagnetic waves. The electrical activity in your heart translates into electromagnetic waves. The electromagnetic field from the heart is so strong that it can be measured as far as 10 feet away. What's even more remarkable is that when you step into the electromagnetic field of another person, your own beat-to-beat variability can be affected. Have you ever walked into a meeting and sensed tension and negativity? It wasn't just because you read everybody's facial expressions and body language. Your heartbeat variability probably changed. Your body can respond to other people's moods physically as well as emotionally. So no matter how positive *you* are, if you are constantly surrounded by negative or hostile people, you will likely find it harder to stay happy.

When Christopher, a 34-year-old actor, joined The Program, he said he felt anxious and worried about everything, even very small things such as whether he had enough dishwasher soap. We helped him learn how to stop frequently throughout the day and do a couple of minutes of slow, deep breathing while he practiced thinking about things he appreciated and loved. After a few weeks of this he found he could quickly switch from feelings of anxiety to feelings of happiness and appreciation. He had learned to turn off his stress response, and just knowing that he had more control of his feelings helped him keep his anxiety in check. He also made an effort to make some new friends and spend more time around happy, upbeat people. He decided that if his heartbeat was going to be affected by the people around him, he wanted the beat-to-beat effect to be a good one.

NUTRITION: SOCIAL EATING

Dining out can be a challenge because the serving sizes are usually big, the food can be tempting but not always healthful, and chefs often slip in high-calorie ingredients you don't know about. But with a few simple strategies, dining out can serve as a nice break from cooking at home without setting you back from your health goals. Here are some strategies to try.

- Eat a healthful snack before you go. You do want to ruin your appetite a little. It's easier to stay in control if you are not ravenous. Don't worry, you'll still enjoy the food.

- Order a salad as an appetizer, with the dressing on the side. Avoid salads with dressing already added, such as tuna salads or potato salad made with mayonnaise. If available, use low-calorie dressing or balsamic vinegar.

- Choose a broth-based soup such as chicken noodle, vegetable, lentil, or bean soup.

- Try to abstain from the bread basket or chip bowl, but if you must indulge, make a firm agreement with yourself that you will have only one roll or ten chips and then have the basket removed from your table.

- The entrée will likely be larger than you need, so you can order an appetizer for your entrée or you can split the entrée with your dining partner. Or you can have the server split it and put half into a doggie bag before he or she brings it to you. Don't be embarrassed to ask for this. If you are going to put part of your entrée in a doggie bag at the end of the meal, it is best to divide the food on your plate in half and put the extra on a separate plate before you start eating your meal. If you try to stop at the halfway mark, you often won't.

- Also, don't be embarrassed to ask for variations of what the restaurant is serving that may be more healthful (such as holding the butter, going light on the cheese, or substituting fruit for french fries). You are the guest. The staff should be eager to please.

- Whether you order an appetizer or an entrée, keep it simple. No gravies, creams, or dishes loaded with high-fat cheese or butter. If there is a sauce, make it tomato-based or wine-based rather than cream- or butter-based. Dishes with names like au gratin, bolognese, hollandaise, and scalloped are all high in fat.

- Ask how the food is prepared. Stay clear of dishes that are battered, breaded, creamed, crispy, or fried. These are code words for high fat.

- Healthful dishes are those that are baked, roasted, steamed, broiled, poached, charbroiled, or grilled.

- Order fish or lean cuts such as skinless chicken.

- Skip dessert. Have some hot tea after the meal. If you decide to have dessert, have fresh fruit, sorbet, or nonfat frozen yogurt. If you must have cake, angel food is your best choice.

What about fast-food restaurants? I'm not encouraging you to eat at fast-food restaurants, but there may be times when you have no choice. Here are some helpful ideas to try.

- Consider ordering a child's portion or order a hamburger with no cheese—hold the mayo. Have them load it up with lots of veggies—lettuce, tomato, onions. Grilled chicken sandwiches are also a good choice if the chicken is grilled and not deep-fried.

- Skip the fries, which are soaked in trans fat. Hello! Those are horrible for you!

- Many fast-food chains offer salads, which can be a great choice but not if they are loaded with cheese or salad dressing. Again, be sure to get the dressing on the side.

- Some fast-food chains are better than others—Subway, in particular, can be a healthful choice.

What about social events? Perhaps you are dining at a friend's house or hosting your own dinner party. Here are some strategies to try.

- If you go to a friend's house, consider bringing something healthy that can help you stay on track, such as a veggie plate, shrimp with cocktail sauce, or a fruit platter. Be sure to check with the host first to make sure it's okay.

- Just as you do before you go to a restaurant, remember to eat a little snack before you leave for the event so you don't arrive ravenous.

- At the event, try keeping one hand busy holding a chilled bottle of water so you are less tempted to use it to pick up too many hors d'ouvres.

- If there is a buffet table, fill your plate as you would at home with lots of veggies, some whole grains, and a protein serving of your choice. Avoid the cheeses, creams, and butters. Go through the line only once. Consider using a small plate.

- Before you go out, decide if you will be having a dessert. If so, limit yourself to one small serving. Do this only if you want to have dessert. If you don't want it, don't feel bad about saying no. You need to learn never to feel bad if you decide not to eat something. Have a prerehearsed line such as "Oh, it looks fabulous! I may have some later, but I'm going to pass right now." Then move on.

- Be careful with alcohol. Alcohol contains seven calories per gram, so it's loaded with calories and has little nutritional value. If you would like it as a treat, you can certainly have one glass, but remember that alcohol can be problematic, not just because of the calories but because of the loss of inhibition that can lead to overeating. Learn to stop after one glass, or skip it altogether.

Practice eating out at a restaurant this week. Before you go, either write down strategies to try that are listed in the suggestions for eating out or feel free to make up your own. Grab a partner. Make it a game to see who can use the most strategies. You can eat a snack before you go, ask the server to modify a dish, have a salad with dressing on the side, separate half your entrée and put it aside, or order an appetizer instead of an entrée. The sky's the limit. Have fun, and remember to use at least a few of these strategies whenever you eat out.

HEALTHY DINING OUT BY CUISINE

ITALIAN FOOD

Quick tips: Skip the bread basket; beware of portion sizes of pasta dishes.

HEALTHY CHOICES	FOODS TO AVOID
Plain bread	Garlic bread
Plain breadsticks	Fried calamari
Salads with dressing on the side	Shrimp scampi
Lentil or minestrone soup	Cheese cannelloni with meat sauce
Baked clams	Spaghetti with meatballs
Fresh seafood	Fettuccine Alfredo
Pasta with red, clam, or wine sauce	Chicken or eggplant parmigiana
Pasta primavera	Cream or white sauces
Skim milk cappuccino	Pastries, cannoli, and tiramisu

FRENCH FOOD

Quick tips: French food is known for containing lots of cheese, cream, and butter; ask how food is prepared and request sauces on the side.

HEALTHY CHOICES	FOODS TO AVOID
French bread	Croissant
Mussels	French onion soup
Bouillabaisse (seafood stew)	En croute (wrapped in pastry)
Coq au vin (chicken stewed in wine)	Potatoes au gratin
Salad Niçoise with the dressing on the side	Beef Bourguignon
Ratatouille	Foie gras
Pot au feu	Quiche Lorraine
Quenelles (steamed fish dumplings)	Chicken cordon bleu
Mixed berries	Hollandaise, Béarnaise, and Béchamel sauces
Sorbet	Buerre blanc (butter sauce)
	Chocolate mousse

GREEK FOOD

Quick tips: This cuisine is noted for using healthy monounsaturated fats, but portion sizes still matter.

HEALTHY CHOICES	FOODS TO AVOID
Pita bread	Saganaki (cheese appetizer)
Hummus	Moussaka
Olives	Falafel in pita
Yogurt and cucumber salad	Pastitsio
Greek salad without the dressing	Gyro
Baba ghanoush	
Dolma (stuffed grape leaves)	
Souvlaki sandwich	
White meat chicken and fish kabobs	

STEAK HOUSE FOOD

Quick tips: Practice portion control; start off with a shrimp cocktail or oyster appetizer; skip high-fat side dishes such as mashed potatoes and creamed spinach; consider ordering fish even though you are at a steak restaurant.

HEALTHY CHOICES	FOODS TO AVOID
Cooked oyster	Bread with butter
Shrimp cocktail	Sour cream
Salads with dressing on the side	Salad with a lot of dressing and cheese
Steak, lean cuts like round or loin with visible fat trimmed off	Mashed potatoes
Steamed vegetables such as broccoli, asparagus, or spinach	Onion rings
Baked potato, no butter	Creamed spinach
	Cheesecake

MEXICAN FOOD

Quick tips: Eat salsa instead of high-fat salad dressings; skip the chips or limit yourself to a portion of ten chips; order food with only one high-fat topping such as cheese, sour cream, or guacamole; fajitas are perfect to split.

HEALTHY CHOICES	FOODS TO AVOID
Soft flour tortillas	Tortilla chips
Sangria	Margaritas
Gazpacho	Nachos
Bean soups	Refried beans
Bean chili	Chorizo (sausage)
Bean, chicken, or seafood fajitas or burritos	Chimichanga (fried burrito)
Salsa	Sour cream
Beans and rice	Guacamole
Taco salad without the shell	Fried ice cream

CHINESE FOOD

Quick tips: Order dishes steamed with sauces on the side; make vegetables the predominant food on your plate; don't be swayed by people wanting to share high-calorie dishes with you; watch out for anything fried or crispy.

HEALTHY CHOICES	FOODS TO AVOID
Clear soups	Fried rice or noodles
Hot-and-sour soup	Fried dumplings
Steamed vegetable, chicken, or shrimp dumplings	Egg rolls or spring rolls
Steamed brown rice	Spare ribs
Stir-fried or steamed chicken or seafood with vegetables	Fried dishes
Chinese vegetables with tofu	Sweet-and-sour dishes
Mu shu pork with no egg	Egg foo yung
Fortune cookies	

JAPANESE FOOD

Quick tips: Generally, Japanese food can be high in salt; ask for low-sodium soy sauce and watch the amount you use; stay away from any items that have "tempura" in their description.

HEALTHY CHOICES	FOODS TO AVOID
Edamame	Tempura (fried food in batter)
Miso or su-udon soup	Tonkatsu (fried pork cutlet)
Sushi and sashimi	Crispy fried noodles
Mizutaki (simmered chicken and vegetables)	
Tossed salad with miso dressing	
Cucumber and seaweed salad	
Steamed gyoza (shrimp dumplings)	
Yosenabe (noodles, seafood, or vegetables in broth)	
Chicken or fish teriyaki	

THAI FOOD

Quick tips: Watch out for dishes with coconut, peanut, or curry sauce; stick with white meat chicken, vegetables, tofu, and stir-fries with the sauce on the side.

HEALTHY CHOICES	FOODS TO AVOID
Lime juice–based salads	Mussaman beef curry
Spring rolls in rice paper	Thai coconut rice
Broth-based soups	Pad thai
Tom yum kung (hot-and-sour soup)	Thai beef salad
Steamed dumplings	Thai coffee or tea
Chicken satay	
Steamed white rice	
Thai seafood salad	
Thai chicken with basil	

INDIAN FOOD

Quick tips: Some terms to learn: *Jhinga* or *paneer tikka* (grilled dishes); *Malai* (means cream); *Makhani* (made in butter); *Naan* (high fat and made with white flour).

HEALTHY CHOICES	FOODS TO AVOID
Chapati or puri bread	Naan bread
House salad	Samosa (fried vegetable or meat patties)
Chicken tikka	Lamb korma (spicy curry)
Tandoori shrimp	Chicken curry
Tandoori chicken without skin	Vegetable fritters
Whole-wheat tandoori roti (without butter)	Lamb biryani
Bean and lentil stew (dal maharani)	Kulfi-faluda or gula jamun (sweet, cream-filled dessert)
Yogurt salad or raita	
Green chutney	
Roasted papade instead of fried papade	
Masala chai	

PIZZERIA FOOD

Quick tips: Ask the pizza maker to go light on the cheese and heavy on the vegetables; fill up first with a side salad with the dressing on the side; choose thin-crust pizzas over thick-crust pizzas.

HEALTHY CHOICES	FOODS TO AVOID
Healthy pizza toppings such as part-skim cheese, feta cheese, vegetables, olives, pineapple, or grilled chicken	Pizza toppings such as extra cheese, several types of cheese, bacon, sausage, or pepperoni
Thin-crust pizza	Deep-dish pizza and Sicilian pizza
Pinch of oregano, basil, or garlic	Breadsticks with butter and garlic bread
Grated parmesan cheese	

SANDWICHES AND SUBS

Quick tips: Ask the sandwich or sub maker to go light on the meat and heavy on the lettuce, onions, tomatoes, and peppers; more healthful condiments include mustard, ketchup, and vinegar; skip the mayo.

HEALTHY CHOICES	FOODS TO AVOID
Turkey breast, smoked turkey, chicken breast, ham, or roast beef	Tuna, chicken, or egg salads with a lot of mayo
Whole-wheat bread	Pastrami and corn beef
Healthy broth-based vegetable and grain soups	Russian dressing
Half or small-size sandwiches	Coleslaw, potato, and macaroni salads
Scoop the dough out of the middle of a big roll or sub	Pasta salad with oil or cream sauce
Salads with light or fat-free dressing	Potato and tortilla chips
Baked chips or pretzels	
Fruit salad	

DINER FOOD

Quick tips: Keep in mind that almost anything can be ordered at a diner all day and prepared the way you like it; don't be afraid to ask for substitutions.

HEALTHY CHOICES	FOODS TO AVOID
Egg-white vegetable omelet	Cheese omelet
Chef's and Greek salad without dressing	BLT (bacon, lettuce, and tomato) sandwich
Grilled chicken salad	Grilled cheese sandwich
Turkey sandwich on whole-wheat bread	Hamburger on bun and french fries
Fruit salad with cottage cheese	Ham and cheese sandwich, grilled
Chicken noodle soup	Tuna, egg, or chicken salad
Turkey and veggie burgers	Rice pudding, pies, cakes, muffins, and danishes
Baked or grilled fish and chicken	
Baked potato	

BUFFET FOOD

Quick tips: Don't go to a buffet on an empty stomach; you don't need to eat your money's worth and leave feeling stuffed; take only small amounts of high-calorie foods; consider ordering a la carte.

HEALTHY CHOICES	FOODS TO AVOID
Vegetables	Salads drenched in dressing
Fruit	Salads prepared with lots of mayonnaise
Lightly dressed salads	Dishes prepared with lots of cheese
Turkey breast	Pasta dishes made with lots of oil and cream sauces
Shrimp cocktail	Muffins
	Pastries
	Desserts

HIGH TEA

Quick tips: Have a small lunch a few hours before your high tea date; this will keep you from being starved and setting yourself up for eating too many goodies; strategize and pick your food mindfully; plan to sip tea rather than fill up on sweets; remember that dinner is only a few hours away.

HEALTHY CHOICES	FOODS TO AVOID
Cucumber, smoked salmon, vegetarian, chicken, tuna, or ham sandwiches	Jam
Fruit and berries	Butter
Bite-size cookies	Cheese
Bite-size pieces of cake	Cream
Mini fruit tarts	Lemon curd
	Large-size scones or other pastries

FAST-FOOD CALORIES

MCDONALD'S

ITEM	CALORIES
Hamburger	250
Cheeseburger	300
Quarter Pounder	410
Quarter Pounder with cheese	510
Big Mac	540
Filet-O-Fish	380
McChicken	360
Premium grilled chicken classic sandwich	420
Premium crispy chicken club sandwich	660
Ranch snack wrap	340
Small fries	230
Large fries	500
Ketchup	15
Chicken McNuggets (four pieces)	190
Chicken McNuggets (ten pieces)	460
Barbecue sauce	50

ITEM	CALORIES
Chicken Selects Premium Breast Strips (five pieces)	630
Asian salad with grilled chicken	300
Premium bacon ranch salad with crispy chicken	370
Premium Caesar salad (without chicken)	90
Premium Caesar salad with grilled chicken	220
Egg McMuffin	300
Sausage McMuffin	450
English muffin	160
Hot fudge sundae	330
Chocolate triple thick shake (16 oz.)	580
Vanilla triple thick shake (16 oz.)	550
Baked hot apple pie	250
Chocolate chip cookie	160

Source: www.mcdonalds.com

SUBWAY

ITEM	CALORIES
6 GRAMS OF FAT OR LESS (Includes lettuce, tomatoes, onions, green peppers, olives, and pickles on Italian white bread)	
Oven roasted chicken breast	310
Roast beef	290
Ham	290
Club	320

ITEM	CALORIES
Veggie delite	230
BMT Biggest-Meatiest-Tastiest	480
SAUCES	
Fat-free sweet onion	40
Fat-free honey mustard	30
Chipotle southwest	100

Source: www.subway.com

DENNY'S

ITEM	CALORIES	ITEM	CALORIES
Side Caesar salad with dressing	362	Hashed browns	200
Deluxe Caesar salad with grilled chicken breast	600	Hashed browns with onions, cheese, and gravy	480
Caesar dressing, 1 oz.	100	Big Texas Chicken Fajita Skillet	1,217
Brown gravy, 1 oz.	13	Classic burger with cheese	836
Ultimate Omelet	670	Country fried potatoes	390
Grilled Chicken Dinner	280	Country scramble	1,038
Carb Watch Burger	625	Banana split	810
Vanilla milk shake	560	Hershey's Chocolate Cake	580

Source: www.dennys.com

STARBUCKS

ITEM	CALORIES	ITEM	CALORIES
BEVERAGES (all calculations are based on the "grande" size)		Caffè Mocha (with whipped cream)	
Caffè Latte		Nonfat	290
Nonfat	130	Whole	360
Whole milk	220	2%	330
2%	190	Soy	320
Soy	170	Cappuccino	
Caffè Mocha (without whipped cream)		Nonfat	80
Nonfat	220	Whole	140
Whole	290	2%	120
2%	260	Soy	110
Soy	250	Coffee of the week	16

ITEM	CALORIES
FOOD (product ingredients vary from store to store)	
Blueberry muffin	520
Blueberry scone	400
Low-fat apple cranberry muffin	250
Low-fat oat fruit scone	320
Lemon pound cake	420

ITEM	CALORIES
Pumpkin loaf	280
Reduced-fat blueberry coffee cake	350
Reduced-fat cinnamon swirl coffee cake	330
Starbucks classic coffee cake	500
Cinnamon swirl	480
Apple fritter	620

Source: www.starbucks.com

JAMBA JUICE

ITEM	CALORIES		
SMOOTHIES	16 OZ.	24 OZ.	32 OZ.
Banana Berry	300	440	600
Caribbean Passion	270	400	520
Chocolate Moo'd	460	660	
Peanut Butter Moo'd	490	800	
Mango-a-go-go	310	450	590
Powerboost		440	570
Protein Berry Workout with Soy	290	440	550
Razzmatazz	300	440	550

ITEM	CALORIES		
JUICES	12 OZ.	16 OZ.	32 OZ.
Carrot	100	130	
Lemonade	300	400	540
Orange	170	220	
Orange/Carrot Banana	150	170	510
Wheatgrass Shot, 1 oz.	5		
Wheatgrass Shot, 2 oz.	10		

Reference: www.dietfacts.com. Source: www.jambajuice.com

MOVIE THEATER SNACKS

ITEM	CALORIES			ITEM	CALORIES
POPCORN	SM	MED	LRG	Starburst Original Fruit Chews (7 oz.)	800
Popped in coconut oil	400	900	1,160		
Popped in coconut oil with "butter" topping	630	1,220	1,640	Milk Duds (4 oz.)	490
				Junior Mints (5½ oz.)	620
Popped in vegetable shortening	360	650	850	M&M's Plain (5½ oz.)	770
CANDY				M&M's Milk Chocolate (5½ oz.)	800
Twizzlers (6 oz.)		560			
Original Fruit Skittles (7 oz.)		770			

Source: Michael F. Jacobson, Ph.D., and Jayne G. Hurley, R.D., *Restaurant Confidential*

There is no doubt that we live in a world where life is busy and filled with endless opportunities for overeating. But this is the world we live in, and it is not going to change. To avoid sacrificing your health, start practicing the strategies just discussed. With a little practice and repetition, you'll find that you can eat out *and* stay healthy!

FITNESS: NUTRITION FOR THE ATHLETE

Whether you are training for a marathon or just pushing yourself to become more physically active, a solid nutrition plan is extremely important. Here are some of the essential things you need to know about a healthy training diet.

FLUIDS

A general rule of thumb is that you should drink a liter or a quart of water for every hour of strenuous exercise. Water is always the best choice for activities that last less than an hour.

For longer activities, you may want to try sports drinks. Sports drinks contain some sugar, which your body needs as fuel. These drinks also replenish the electrolytes you lose during heavy sweating. You can save money and make your own sports drink:

1   Dissolve a tablespoon of sugar and a pinch of salt into a tablespoon of orange juice or 2 tablespoons of lemon juice.

2   Add 7.5 ounces of cold water, stir or shake, and enjoy!

Be sure to check the color of your urine to make sure you are hydrated. Dark-colored urine indicates dehydration. If you are fully hydrated, you will have pale yellow urine.

Vitamins and Supplements

Do you need extra vitamins and supplements? I don't recommend lots of supplements because they are expensive and have not been shown in randomized well-designed studies to make any significant difference. I do, however, recommend a daily multivitamin to be sure that you meet all of your nutritional needs.

Food

As far as food is concerned, you will want to increase the carbohydrates in your diet to about 60 percent of your total calories. Carbohydrates (which are broken down into sugar) are an athlete's best energy source. When you exercise, your body first taps into the sugar in your bloodstream; it then uses the sugar stored in your liver and muscles. These stores are called glycogen stores. After about two hours of strenuous activity, your blood sugar and glycogen stores are all used up. When this happens, you can't perform at a high level, much less at all. This loss of sugar is what is behind the "hitting the wall" phenomenon in marathoners who do not take in extra fuel when running.

What if you are trying to build muscles by strength training? Consuming protein supplements will not in and of itself build muscle. It's strength training that builds muscle. As I've said before, any excess protein that is not used will just be converted into fat. It's true that you need enough protein in your diet to provide protein building blocks for that new muscle, but most American diets provide more than enough protein. If you are doing major strength training, you will probably be consuming more calories and therefore increasing your protein naturally without supplements.

As far as the fats in your diet are concerned, you don't need to concentrate too much on this area except to know that the bulk of your fats should be coming from mainly unsaturated fats. No more than 10 percent of your fats should be coming from saturated fats, and ideally you aren't eating any trans fats. This means that if you are taking in more protein, you need to find other ways of doing this than through hamburgers and steaks, both of which are high in saturated fat.

Healthful eating helps you maintain your strength, flexibility, and endurance. The best diet for an athlete is one that is varied, moderate, and balanced. It should be high in carbohydrates with enough protein, vitamins, minerals, and fluids—and not too much fat. A high-performance diet is appropriate for all physically active people, not just those training for sporting events and competitions.

Training for and participating in a big athletic event can be exhilarating and empowering. Don't dismiss this sort of thing as something only jocks can do. One of my patients, Sam, is a computer engineer who never really participated in sports in the past. When Sam started to exercise eight months ago, he began by walking one mile around his neighborhood. Before long, he had worked up to three miles. He then started to run. It was more of a walk-run. After several months of running, he decided he wanted to train for a marathon. At first I thought he was pushing too fast too soon, but he proved me wrong. He started running three miles three times a week and one long run every weekend. At first the long run was five miles, and every weekend he increased the mileage by two miles. On the days he did not run, he simply stretched and did a little weight lifting. A couple of weeks before the marathon, he ran twenty miles, and then he consciously cut back on the running, only going on short runs a few times a week. He easily ran the twenty-six-mile-marathon. The week after the marathon, two work colleagues came up to him privately to tell him how impressed they were and ask how he had done it. Both had seen how exhilarating and empowering this experience had been for Sam and they wanted a piece of that, too. Remember, though, that you don't need to run an actual marathon to share in these benefits; it's simply about exercise, pushing yourself, having goals, and seeing yourself follow through.

On your mark, get set, *go*!

LEARN IT!

- Mood chemicals in your brain influence the way you feel, but you can influence these chemicals by how you think and how you live.

- The major mood chemicals are **serotonin**, **norepinephrine**, and **dopamine**; the levels of these chemicals are often low in depression and anxiety.

- The physical nerve networks in your brain influence how you feel and respond to things. You can physically restructure your brain's nerve pathways to provide alternate paths of thought for a given situation, which can help a lot with your mood.

- Exercise not only increases mood chemicals, it actually promotes physical restructuring within the brain.

- You *can* remain healthy even if you go to a lot of social events or eat out at restaurants.

- Nutritional advice for the athlete is not significantly different from that which everyone should be following.

PERSONALIZE IT!

This week, work on your Exercising Brain.

Exercise changes both the function and the physical structure of the brain. It increases numerous chemicals in both the brain and the body that elevate mood, decrease stress, and increase mental alertness. Physical exercise also significantly increases brain activity, facilitating learning and memory. Exercise is your biggest ally in health *and* in behavior change because it optimizes the performance of both the body and the brain.

Here are some examples of how people in The Program have personalized this brain principle and put it into action.

- Tony O., a 61-year-old business owner, had always had issues with anxiety. He described himself as "tightly wound," and he frequently worried about things that never materialized. When he started exercising regularly, he found himself dramatically more relaxed and happy. He made sure he exercised before any big meeting that required him to be mentally alert and creative because it helped so much.

- Chloe A., a 21-year-old college student, had suffered from low-level depression her whole life, but when school became particularly stressful she decided she needed to do something. She began counseling and was given a low-dose antidepressant. She began to run consistently. The regular exercise helped her mood significantly, but what she found even more surprising was that she was also more alert in class and learned material in school more easily.

LIVE IT!

- Review last week's goals and create this week's short-term goals.

- Review the top ten Happiness Strategies discussed in this chapter. Are there any you would like to try?

- Practice eating out at a restaurant this week.

- Review your food log and exercise log. How are you doing? Do you see any patterns? Are you eating too little during the day and too heavily in the evening? Are you eating a 4 P.M. snack so that you are less likely to overeat at dinner?

- Consider training for an athletic event. You can look on the Internet to find events in your local area.

CONQUERING ADDICTION

Whether you think you can or whether you think you can't, you're right.

—HENRY FORD

THIS CHAPTER IS FOR EVERYONE, not just for those who are addicted to something. What may seem surprising to you at first is that the physiology of attention, motivation, and even happiness involves the same circuits and chemicals that are involved in addiction.

Somewhere around 7 to 8 percent of the general U.S. population has tried illegal drugs at some point in their lives. There has been a dramatic rise in American drug addiction since 1960. No one is immune. We see it in men and women, young and old. We see it in all races, through all socioeconomic levels. Addiction knows no boundaries.

While the word *addiction* may make you think of smoking or alcohol, cocaine or methamphetamine, there are many other things besides these traditional substances that can trigger addictive physiology—things like gambling, sex, food, even playing video games. All of these behaviors can generate high levels of dopamine, a feel-good chemical, in a couple of distinct areas of the brain known as pleasure centers.

Here's how addiction works. Deep in the brain, there are areas called the nucleus accumbens and ventral tegmental area, also known as the "pleasure centers." You get a pleasurable sensation from the release of dopamine when this area is activated. Some people have a much more intense reaction to a given stimulus than another person by generating more dopamine.

Dopamine feels good and captures your attention, but too high a level can cause hallucinations or distorted thinking, and when high levels of dopamine are released on a repeated basis, larger and larger amounts are needed to have the same effect, as the receptors on the nerve cell membrane become less and less responsive. This phenomenon is known as *tolerance.* After a while, not only does it take higher levels of dopamine to have the same effect; even normal levels of dopamine don't feel as if they are enough anymore. Because the normal levels feel low, all the brain can think about is how to get the dopamine into a range that will feel normal again. Some drugs, such as methamphetamine, trigger this physiology quite quickly. People often become addicted to this drug after one or two exposures. What about other drugs? They all differ in their ability to cause addiction, and people also differ in how easily they can become addicted.

Let me give you an example of how people differ in addiction physiology by going over some interesting rat studies. In one study, rats were hooked up to electrical stimulation circuits where they were able to activate their pleasure centers as often as they liked. There were three genetically distinct rats. One type of rat, the Lewis rat, was striking in its motivation to activate its pleasure centers. These rats were so obsessed with the task of pleasure activation that they stopped eating and drinking and sleeping, and after about five days they died. Another kind of rat, the Sprague-Dawley rat, exhibited a medium response. Although these rats spent quite a bit of their day stimulating their pleasure centers, they did stop to eat, drink, and sleep. Finally, there was a third group of rats called the Fischer rats. These little guys weren't much interested in stimulating their pleasure centers. They tried it a few times but seemed fairly uninterested. Human beings also demonstrate variability in their desire to activate their pleasure centers. People also vary in the types of things that will activate their pleasure centers. For example, one person may be more vulnerable to becoming addicted to gambling or video games, while another person may be more vulnerable to shopping, sex, or eating addictions.

Genetic variations can increase the likelihood of a person becoming addicted. Many alcoholics have a genetic alteration that reduces their number of dopamine receptors, thereby lowering the brain's ability to perceive dopamine. This gene variation is called the D2R2 allele. Although 25 percent of the general population has this allele, 75 percent of severe alcoholics have it, as do 50 to 80 percent of those addicted to drugs! The D2R2 allele is also linked to depression and ADD.

Fifty percent of those who struggle with ADD, or attention deficit disorder, also struggle with substance abuse. Medications given for ADD or ADHD raise dopamine levels. Exercise, as I've mentioned before, is also a very effective way to raise dopamine levels.

Let me be clear that if you have a genetic predisposition to addiction, it does not necessarily mean that you will have a problem with addiction. You, and only you, have the final say in that. What it does mean is that if you are exposed to certain addictive substances or behaviors, you will run a higher risk of becoming addicted than would someone who didn't have that gene. Likewise, if you don't have any genetic predisposition, it certainly does not mean you cannot become addicted; it simply decreases the likelihood.

Of course, the pleasure center has an evolutionary purpose. It did not evolve just so you could get some kicks. The pleasure center, when stimulated, sends dopamine to the prefrontal cortex, where decisions are made and impulses are suppressed. Your prefrontal cortex needs to be stimulated enough through this reward system to be motivated to do something; otherwise it isn't very cooperative. The prefrontal cortex depends on the reward center to tell it what it should focus on, to make it do things that require delayed gratification. For example in ADD, as already mentioned, dopamine levels are low. People with ADD have trouble with delayed gratification. They have trouble maintaining their focus, and they want instant rewards. As I've also said, ADD is treated with medications that increase dopamine, therefore increasing one's focus and attention.

Exercise is a wonderful way to boost dopamine levels, too. It also boosts the level of endocannabinoids—a natural marijuanalike brain chemical that is pleasant, calming, and thought to be the cause of "runner's high"—in your brain. If you have issues with addiction or have in the past, I strongly recommend getting into a regular exercise program. Because exercise dramatically increases dopamine, it lowers withdrawal symptoms. For smokers, just five minutes of intense exercise can reduce cravings. In drug rehabilitation programs, those who engage in exercise are twice as likely to remain drug-free.

But exercise isn't the only way you can elevate your dopamine levels naturally. Lots of things naturally stimulate the release of dopamine, such as being with friends and lovers, curling up with a good book, listening to music, watching a sunset, collecting baseball cards, really anything you enjoy! Sex, incidentally, increases dopamine levels by 100 percent. This is nature's way of making sure you reproduce so that you will pass on your genes. Not surprisingly, all of the things that promote survival are associated with pleasure center activation: sex, food, love, social connections, and physical movement, to name a few. This is why it is important, when creating a healthy routine, that you also try to make it fun. Otherwise you aren't likely to do it for very long.

What excites and motivates you? Perhaps you are very social and would enjoy starting a competition around healthy behavior at work. Or maybe you would like to train for a competition. Do you like rewards? Think about what you could do to motivate your healthy behavior. Robin, for example, wanted a pearl necklace, so every week that she kept working at her new healthy lifestyle, she put away money equal to one pearl on the necklace. She did, by the way, eventually earn the whole necklace. Renee, on the other hand, had some favorite comedy shows she loved to watch, so she set up her treadmill so she could watch her shows while she ran (and laughed).

MEDICATIONS USED IN ADDICTION

- One effective medication used in smoking cessation is **Zyban,** known generically as bupropion. This medication produces higher dopamine levels in order to avoid the precipitous drop a smoker experiences when he or she stops smoking.

- A newer medication for smoking cessation is **Chantix,** known generically as varenicline. It activates the nicotinic receptors that cause the release of dopamine, but it does so only partially. It provides a small, steady release of dopamine while blocking the usual rush of dopamine that smoking typically provides. Thus, there is no positive reinforcement.

- **Vivitrol** and **Revia,** known generically as naltrexone, are both medications for treating alcohol that block alcohol from binding to the opioid receptors that activate dopamine. This medication blocks the positive reinforcement of alcohol.

- A new medication, **Acamprosate,** is being used to treat alcohol addiction. Its molecular structure is similar to that of glutamate. Acamprosate slows the release of glutamate. (Glutamate can be too stimulating and overwhelming for the brain.) By slowing its release, one may feel less inclined to calm the brain with alcohol.

- **Baclofen,** a muscle relaxant, stimulates production of the inhibitor GABA. GABA's role is the opposite of glutamate's. Baclofen appears to reduce the cravings for several different addictive substances.

- **Topiramate** is an antiseizure medication that appears to increase GABA levels and reduce cravings for addictive substances. In one (manufacturer-supported) research study, 370 adults with alcohol dependence were randomized to Topiramate (up to 300 milligrams daily) or a placebo for fourteen weeks, and Topiramate significantly reduced alcohol consumption.

- **Rimonabant** is a medication that blocks the cannabanoid receptors (the same receptors stimulated by marijuana). Our bodies naturally produce a marijuanalike chemical known as endocannabinoid. Blockage of this receptor appears to decrease cravings for food, nicotine, and alcohol. When it came up for FDA review in 2007, it was not approved for use in the United States because of psychiatric side effects.

Alcohol

One question I am asked a lot is whether drinking alcohol is healthful or unhealthful. First, if you find it hard to stop once you start drinking, you are better off not having anything to drink. Also, you should not drink if you have liver problems. For many people, occasional alcohol consumption can fit fine into a healthy lifestyle. Wine, in particular, in modest amounts can decrease the risk of heart disease. But remember, it does need to be a modest amount.

Women should not have more than one drink a day on the average; more than this increases mortality and raises the risk of health issues such as breast cancer. Men should not have more than two on the average; more than that leads to an increase in mortality. A serving size of alcohol is 4 ounces for wine; that's smaller than many people's wine serving. It's impossible to tell you how much of a wineglass is equal to 4 ounces because wineglasses vary so much in size. Fill a measuring cup with water to the half-cup mark and pour it into the wineglass you typically use. That is what your serving size should be. An equivalent serving of beer is 12 ounces (a typical beer can or bottle) and hard liquor is 1½ ounces (one ounce equals a shot). You can experiment with different ways of keeping your alcohol portions limited. For example, you can mix alcohol with club soda, a diet soft drink, tonic water, tomato juice, or reduced-sugar fruit juice to dilute the alcohol content.

Smoking

From *The Washington Post,* February 7, 2008:

> *Tobacco use killed 100 million people worldwide in the twentieth century and could kill one billion people in the twenty-first unless governments act now to dramatically reduce it, the World Health Organization said in a report Thursday.*

By now you are well aware that smoking dramatically accelerates the risk of developing plaque in your blood vessels, and greatly increasing the risk of heart attacks and strokes. Of course, it is also very destructive to your cell's DNA and promotes lots of different kinds of cancers. Smoking also accelerates the aging process. *It is actually the number one lifestyle-related cause of death in our country.*

I know that giving up smoking can be really tough, but I encourage you to consider giving it a try. In preparation, learn as much as you can from other people who have stopped successfully. I also suggest you create a good support network, as this will really help. There are smoking hotlines and all sorts of programs available, and you can also work with a friend, a loved one, or a health professional. There are many smoking cessation aids available now as well. There are nicotine replacement treatments (patches and gum) and even inhaling devices and nasal spray. There are also temporary medications that can increase your odds of getting off nicotine. They work partly by replenishing the dopamine levels in your brain so you don't experience such big withdrawal symptoms.

Talk to your doctor about what is available. Start a good exercise program. Exercise drives up your dopamine levels, which crash temporarily when you stop smoking. Focus on healthy nutrition. Stress management techniques and adequate amounts of sleep will also help. Smoking cessation is the best thing you can do to get healthier.

TOP TWENTY TIPS FOR SMOKING CESSATION

1   **Make a list of all the reasons you want to quit smoking** and keep this list close at hand, especially during the first three months of quitting.

2   **List potential challenges** you may encounter along the way and create a game plan for how you might handle these situations if and when they occur.

3   **Consider meeting with your doctor** to discuss whether you might be a good candidate for nicotine replacement or anticraving medications such as Chantix or Zyban. Antismoking aids can more than double your chances of success. If you decide to stop smoking cold turkey, know that the first seventy-two hours are the hardest. It does get easier. Really.

4   **Decide on a quit date** no more than two weeks in advance. Write it down. Even consider creating a written contract with yourself.

5   **Don't forget to include rewards in your plan**—maybe a small reward after the first twenty-four hours, then the first week, then the first month, and so on. Include this in your contract.

6   **Tell all your friends and family that you will be quitting** on the quit date you have selected. They can help keep you accountable and can also be a great source of support during some of the difficult times ahead.

7   **Set up a partner or buddy to work with or join a support group.** Having a solid social network to rely on is extremely helpful in smoking cessation. There is a free hotline provided by the American Cancer Society that provides telephone-based support. The number is 1-877-937-7848.

8 **Expect to have mood swings during the first few weeks.** Things will definitely get better, but go easy on yourself during this time. Avoid taking on any high-stress projects.

9 **Try to fill your days with projects you find enjoyable.** Though you don't want to take on any high-stress projects, you do want to stay busy.

10 **Change your environment to minimize smoking cues.** Remove ashtrays from your home and office. Minimize your contact with people who are smoking. Stay away from places where people are actively smoking.

11 **Pay attention to how much alcohol you drink** because alcohol tends to decrease inhibition which can lead to relapse.

12 **Exercise daily.** This is one of the most helpful things you can do to stop smoking. Exercise helps reduce stress, elevates mood, and minimizes your chances of weight gain. It also elevates your dopamine levels so you have fewer withdrawal symptoms and cravings.

13 **Be very mindful of both diet and daily exercise.** While weight gain (of 5 to 10 pounds) is common when you stop smoking, it is not inevitable. A combination of exercise and careful attention to your diet not only helps keep your weight stable, it can even allow for weight loss.

14 **Drink plenty of fluids throughout the day.** Part of the reason for this is that it will fulfill some of that compulsive desire to put something in your mouth. Also, it will help keep you full so you are less likely to nibble on snacks that could contribute to weight gain. Finally, there are hundreds of different chemicals that have entered your body through smoking, so drinking lots of fluid helps flush these toxins out of your system.

15 **Get plenty of sleep.** Insufficient sleep leads to higher stress levels and increases the likelihood of relapse.

16 **Don't think that "just one puff" will be okay.** Even one puff will greatly enhance your chance of relapse.

17 **Be realistic about the process.** Giving up smoking does involve a loss that can feel substantial. Many people feel as if they are giving up their best friend when they stop smoking, a "friend" they always turned to when times were tough. But keep reminding yourself that this "friend" is one that can and will kill you.

18 **Never let your guard down completely.** Although the more time that goes by, the easier it is to remain smoke-free, be aware that the future will bring moments of weakness and temptation.

19 **Savor the positive results,** such as a higher level of self-confidence from seeing yourself succeed in this challenge, the ability to breathe more easily during exercise, diminished cough, and no more smoker's breath. Relish your markedly improved health status. Count the money you have saved by no longer having to support this habit.

20 **Stay positive. Believe in yourself.** There is no question that smoking cessation can be hard, but millions of people have successfully stopped smoking, and you can too.

Smoking Cessation Aids

Nicotine replacement therapy is designed to prevent and treat the withdrawal symptoms experienced by people when they stop smoking. These withdrawal symptoms are what 70 to 90 percent of smokers say is the sole reason they don't quit. There are many different forms of nicotine replacement, which are listed below. *Do not use nicotine replacement treatments and continue to smoke at the same time.*

Nicotine Gum

Nicotine gum comes in 2- and 4-milligram doses and can be obtained without prescription. The 4-milligram dose is appropriate for heavier smokers, those who smoke more than one pack a day. Chew the gum slowly until you taste the peppery flavor, then tuck the gum against your cheek; chew and tuck intermittently over thirty minutes to allow the nicotine to be absorbed fully through your cheek's mucous membrane. You can chew up to twenty pieces a day, tapering off over a three-month period to wean yourself from nicotine entirely. Do not eat or drink within fifteen minutes of chewing, or it will diminish the nicotine absorption.

Advantages: Fast acting; avoids the skin irritation that can occur with patches; provides more flexibility to match replacement therapy with cravings.

Disadvantages: Sore throat, mouth sores, jaw discomfort, damage to dentures or dental prostheses, racing heartbeat, headache, nausea, insomnia.

Nicotine Patch

Available both over the counter and by prescription, the nicotine patch provides a steady, continuous level of nicotine throughout the day. The nicotine is absorbed through the skin. You replace the patch daily, applying it to a nonhairy area of your body below your neck but above your waist. The arm is a common location. You can try a sixteen-hour patch if you are a light to average smoker but should use a twenty-four-hour patch if you are a heavy smoker and have intense cravings in the morning. Note, however, that the twenty-four-hour patch is more likely to cause insomnia and skin irritation than the sixteen-hour patch. Both the twenty-four- and sixteen-hour patches are offered in different strengths; use the higher strength for the first four to six weeks, then wean yourself to the lower doses over the next four to six weeks.

The goal is to taper off the nicotine entirely over a three-month period. You want to taper off the nicotine because although taking in nicotine this way is arguably better for your health than smoking, it is still not entirely benign, as it raises blood pressure and puts stress on the heart. Nicotine replacement is meant as a short-term measure to get you past the toughest phase of tobacco cessation.

Advantages: Slow absorption helps to reduce nicotine side effects; steady levels help prevent sudden nicotine withdrawal that can lead to intense cravings.

Disadvantages: Insomnia, especially with the twenty-four-hour patch, skin irritation, headache, nausea.

NICOTINE LOZENGES

Nicotine lozenges are the newest form of nicotine replacement and are available over the counter. As with nicotine gum, the doses are 2 and 4 milligrams. The lozenge is designed to be sucked until dissolved, not chewed or swallowed whole. No food or drink is to be taken while sucking the lozenge or within fifteen minutes of finishing it in order to maximize nicotine absorption.

Advantages: Fast acting; as with nicotine gum, the lozenge allows you to have more control over dosing.

Disadvantages: Sore throat, headache, insomnia, nausea, gas.

NICOTINE INHALER

Introduced in 1998, nicotine inhalers are available only by prescription. The nicotine is delivered through a plastic tube shaped like a cigarette, which has a nicotine cartridge within it. When you puff on the inhaler, the cartridge releases a nicotine vapor. Unlike other inhalers, which deliver the medication to the lungs, the nicotine inhaler delivers most of the nicotine vapor to the mouth, where it is absorbed through the mucous membranes. No more than sixteen cartridges a day should be used; taper off over a three-month period.

Advantages: Because this form of therapy is so similar to smoking, some smokers find this the most comforting form of replacement when they are experiencing withdrawal.

Disadvantages: This is the most expensive form of nicotine replacement. Side effects include headache, nausea, and insomnia.

NICOTINE NASAL SPRAY

Available only by prescription, the nicotine nasal spray is very effective and offers immediate relief from withdrawal symptoms. You should wean yourself from using the nasal spray over a three-month period.

Advantages: Quick, potent, easy to use.

Disadvantages: Nasal irritation, runny nose, watery eyes, sore throat. People with a history of allergies or asthma or nasal polyps should use a different nicotine replacement therapy. Side effects are headache, nausea, and insomnia.

BUPROPION (ZYBAN)

Bupropion is a prescription antidepressant that reduces nicotine withdrawal symptoms. It does not contain nicotine but rather elevates dopamine levels in the brain. Dopamine levels plummet when smokers abruptly stop smoking, and it is this sudden drop in dopamine that results in the cravings ex-smokers experience early on. The usual dose of bupropion is 150 to 300 milligrams per day.

Advantages: May be used alone or in combination with nicotine replacement therapy; may promote appetite suppression.

Disadvantages: May cause insomnia or jitteriness; should not be used by anyone with a history of seizures, head trauma, heavy alcohol use, or anorexia.

Varenicline (Chantix)

Varenicline is a newer medication designed specifically to help people quit smoking. It targets the nicotine receptors, so it not only reduces withdrawal symptoms, it also diminishes the pleasurable physical effects of smoking. Studies suggest that this medication can more than double your chances of smoking cessation, and some studies have found it more effective than bupropion.

Advantages: Well tolerated and effective.

Disadvantages: The combination of nicotine replacement with varenicline may be potentially associated with more nicotine side effects, although the use of both together is not contraindicated. Side effects include headache, nausea, insomnia, and possible mood changes.

Toby, a 49-year-old marketing executive from New York, joined The Program to better control his weight and diabetes, but in talking to him it became clear he drank too much alcohol. Toby knew he had a problem, too. His father and brother were both alcoholics, and although he liked his two (or three or four) drinks when he got home from work, he admitted he found it hard to stop. Toby went to Alcoholic Anonymous. He developed a strong support group there, found a sponsor, and stopped drinking entirely. He had one relapse in the first three months, but that was it. He has been sober ever since. He took antidepressants for a year to treat the depression he was also struggling with, and he also became an avid runner. The exercise helped him tremendously, calming him down, lifting his mood, and increasing his productivity.

Sharon had a different kind of addiction. Now a 36-year-old assistant to a car dealership owner, she had been a methamphetamine addict since the age of 12. The turning point for her was the day her 18-month-old-daughter was taken from her care while Sharon served time in jail. It was not clear that Sharon would ever get her daughter back. She had to prove herself to the courts first.

At that point Sharon had been addicted to drugs for nineteen years. What was the likelihood that she could change? The answer is simple. Everyone has the ability to change when they want it badly enough, and Sharon wanted to have her daughter back more than anything in the world. Sharon stopped taking drugs and underwent random drug testing for a year; she went through a rehabilitation program, and she joined a support group. She got a minimum-wage job (which was not easy due to her criminal record), and she found a place to live where she could safely raise her daughter. She took medication for anxiety and depression. In addition to medication, she started running.

Sharon was in terrible physical shape when she started, and she began by walking, but in a couple of months she was running. She found that daily vigorous exercise was extremely helpful to her mood. She also found it crucial to maintain structure within her day. Order in her life, coupled with a good sleep schedule, helped her maintain a more stable mood. To this day, five years later, she remains drug-free and has been reunited with her daughter, who, I'm happy to say, is thriving beautifully.

NUTRITION: EMOTIONAL EATING

Emotional eating is extremely common among both men and women. Most people engage in it at least occasionally. Some people do it when they feel stressed or frustrated. Others do it when they are bored, sad, tired, or lonely. The truth is, food can help you feel better. It can calm you down when you feel stressed, and it can lift your mood. Unfortunately, it can also cause you to gain weight. What is the best way to deal with this issue?

First, you should know that emotional eating, while it won't help you reach your health goals, makes perfect physiologic sense. I'm going to review this for you because I think that understanding the process can be helpful in taking the first step toward overcoming it.

As we've already discussed, research studies have used functional MRI and PET scans to study the areas of the brain that activate during stress. These studies have identified the amygdala, deep in the brain, as a key player. The same studies have also looked at what happens to the brain when people eat. The findings are quite interesting.

It turns out that the amygdala does not fire while you are eating. It appears that the stress response turns off when food is put into your system probably because the introduction of food forces blood flow from your muscles to your gut. During stress, remember, blood is shunted away from the gut to the muscles, so when you force blood in the opposite direction, this appears to serve as a negative feedback signal to the brain. The brain hears the message "All clear! No life-threatening emergency happening here! I'm eating!"

In a follow-up study done at a different institution, researchers set out to confirm these findings. Sure enough, particularly when patients ate high-fat or high-sugar foods, they experienced a drop in cortisol, epinephrine, and norepineprine; there was also a decrease in the activity of the sympathetic nervous system. Of course, the drop doesn't last forever, but this does explain a lot about the incentives for emotional eating.

Another study, published in 2001, found that people who produced a high level of cortisol in response to stress tended to eat more in stressful situations than in nonstressful situations. The high cortisol producers also tended to consume more sweet foods than those who produced less cortisol. As with stress, depression elevates cortisol levels. Many people tend to eat more during times of sadness or depression as well as stress.

A British survey found that 63 percent of the adults surveyed had lower self-esteem when they felt they were overweight but 52 percent of these same people felt better instantly when they ate chocolate. Chocolate, in fact, stimulates dopamine release in the nucleus accumbens, the pleasure center, and causes mood elevation in many people almost immediately after eating it.

Now, don't misinterpret what I'm saying. I'm not encouraging you to have a brownie the next time your boss yells at you, but I do want you to understand why you may be tempted to eat when you are feeling stressed. Even though it does make you feel better temporarily, you need to see emotional eating for what it is—a short-term fix. The key to controlling this response is to develop alternative strategies that will help you deal with your feelings and moods.

In addition to the physiologic response to food, most people have a psychological association with it. For most of us, food represents love, nurturing, and comfort. Often, there are cultural, ethnic, and religious associations with food. For people all over the world, eating is an integral part of socializing and participating in life.

Binge eating appears to be related to the addiction physiology just discussed. Just as with addiction, some people are more susceptible to binge eating than others. For people who are like the Fisher rats and are not particularly affected by stimulation of the pleasure centers, there is usually no problem with addiction. But for those who are more like the Lewis rats, which just can't get enough dopamine, know that there are all kinds of new treatments, therapies, and medications now available to help kick bad habits. Paying attention to the dopamine level in your brain might make a big difference whether you binge-eat.

How can you enjoy food, then, without letting it assume a larger role than it should have in your life? How can you break away from using food as a type of self-medication? Here are some strategies to try.

- Every time you want to eat, use the HALT method to make sure you are really hungry. Ask yourself: Am I Hungry? Am I Angry? Am I Lonely? Am I Tired?

- Have a list of distracting activities to do when you feel a craving to eat. For example, call a friend, take a walk, work on a hobby or project, take a warm bath, listen to music—do anything that brings you joy or soothes you.

- Don't keep your trigger foods, the ones you crave, on hand. They become too big a temptation in vulnerable times.

- Wait fifteen minutes before giving in to a craving. A craving typically lasts two to twelve minutes, so if you can distract yourself or change the setting, the craving will pass 90 percent of the time.

- Take some slow, deep breaths to shut off the stress response.

- If you are prone to eating under stress, do as much as you can to manage your stress. This includes getting regular exercise, eating regular meals, and getting enough sleep.

- You may find relief from yoga or meditation.

- If you have a relapse, analyze your behavior and learn from it. Make a plan for the next time you have cravings.

- If you really have difficulty preventing emotional eating, try to limit the damage by committing to a course of action before it happens. Some people are able to allow themselves a small amount of their favorite food; some people, however, are best served by completely avoiding a particular trigger food since they are not able to eat just a small amount of it. If this is the case with you, decide in advance on the specific occasions when you will indulge yourself in a little of your favorite food.

- Sometimes it helps to consult a counselor who can help you work through any emotional issues you may be experiencing.

- If you find yourself in the middle of a binge and cannot control yourself, try ruining the food so you can't eat it. Run water over it or throw it down the garbage disposal.

The trick to overcoming emotional eating is not to depend solely on the mind-over-matter approach. Come up with concrete, realistic strategies that you can use in situations that typically drive you to eat. Whatever ideas you come up with, it is important to practice them over and over. Eventually, this will pay off as your brain gets used to substituting new behaviors for these same old emotional triggers. And remember, it's always easier to create a new habit than to break an old one, so wherever you can, think of new habits that make the old behavior more difficult to do.

Think about whether you participate in emotional eating. Most people do to some extent, so don't feel bad if the answer is yes. What kinds of things trigger you to eat? Are they actual emotions, such as anger, loneliness, frustration, stress, or sadness—or is there a certain time of day, such as when you come home from work? Or does an activity trigger you to eat, such as when you are watching television or doing your homework? First identify these triggers. Then think of a few alternative strategies you could try in place of eating. Review the strategies in this chapter that have worked for other people if you need ideas. And remember, whenever you have a food craving, try waiting fifteen minutes to see if the craving will pass.

Think about whether you binge eat. Do you tend to eat until you are physically uncomfortable and feel out of control? Do you do so secretly? If so, you may want to consult with a counselor or dietitian who is trained in binge eating. For some people, eating is a true addiction, with the same addiction physiology as drugs, alcohol, or cigarettes, so it should be addressed in the same way.

Tina is 27 and suffers from binge eating. It started when she was a teenager, when she got into a routine of eating little during the day but letting herself get out of control at night. She would eat large quantities of high-fat and high-sugar foods. Sometimes she would mix together flour, butter, and sugar to eat if there was nothing in the cupboard that appealed to her. Sometimes she would wake up in the middle of the night, go to the food cupboard, and eat full loaves of bread or containers of ice cream.

It took far longer than the twelve weeks of The Program to overcome this behavior, but through counseling, exercise, and a concerted effort to eat small, frequent meals, she has been able to turn her behavior around slowly over several years. She has become quite skilled at reducing stress with deep breathing and mental imagery, and she is very good at reframing a situation in which she finds herself upset. When she comes home from work, she relaxes by knitting, playing music, and talking to friends on the phone, but even after several years of good control, she sometimes finds herself having a binge. When this happens, she has learned to destroy the food by washing it down the garbage disposal. She then brushes her teeth and jumps rope until she is exhausted. This almost always ends the episode.

FITNESS: PREVENTING SPORTS INJURIES

All those who play a sport should realize that they are at risk of injury. Sports injuries occur most frequently due to trauma, poor conditioning, or muscle or joint overuse. Let's run through the major factors involved in injury prevention.

First, always warm up before you exercise. Research shows that cold muscles and tendons are more prone to injury because they do not stretch well and therefore tear more easily. During your warm-up, muscle fibers and tendons can warm up simply because your body temperature increases. Basically, you can do whatever activity you plan on doing, but do it at about half the intensity for the first five minutes.

Traditionally, it was thought that a warm-up should include stretching muscles and tendons to prevent them from possible strain that occurs with high levels of function. But research has suggested that stretching immediately before exercise does not prevent overuse or acute injuries. A regular program of stretching, however, can.

Proper rest and nutrition are not only necessary for optimal performance, they are important in preventing injury as well. Hydration is also essential when participating in a sport. Dehydration of as little as 2 percent can affect physical performance, which then increases the odds of becoming injured.

Allow ample time to prepare for competition. There should be a slow buildup of intensity to reach peak performance. Too much, too soon is often the cause of injury from overuse. An increase of about 10 percent per week is recommended to prepare your body properly for the activity and prevent injury.

Take lessons and invest in the right equipment. Even if you have been playing a sport for a long time, lessons or coaching is a worthwhile investment. Proper form and technique reduce your chances of developing an overuse injury. Wear shoes appropriate for the sport you are playing, and replace them as needed. Use properly fitted equipment, including safety equipment.

Cross train. Vary your activities so that you are regularly using different muscle groups. This helps to avoid overuse injuries in muscles, tendons, and joints. Balance is the key when training for any sport. Always strive for balance in strength, flexibility, diet, rest time, and frequency and intensity of training sessions.

Plantar Fasciitis

Plantar fasciitis is the most common injury of the foot. It is an inflammation of the connective tissue extending from the calcaneus, or heel bone, to the metatarsals at the ball of your foot. Repetitive use from prolonged walking or running leads to small tears in the fascia, resulting in scarring and pain. This can cause the feet to be stiff in the morning with pain on the undersurface of the feet when walking. To treat or prevent plantar fasciitis, it is important that you have supportive, cushioned shoes. You can buy inserts for shoes to improve support and cushioning. In severe cases, physical therapy and orthotics are necessary, but in most cases complete recovery is possible simply with better foot support, rest, ice, and sometimes a short course of anti-inflammatories. You can also do three simple stretching exercises at home to speed resolution and prevent recurrence. Stretching is most effective if you do it several times a day.

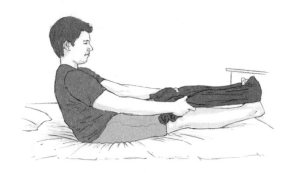

For the first stretch, keep a towel next to your bed, and before you get up in the morning, use the towel to stretch your calf. Hold both ends of the towel and place the middle of it over the ball of your foot as you sit up in bed. Pull back on the ends of the towel until you feel a stretch in the back of your calf. Hold for 30 seconds.

For the second stretch, stand with one foot in front of the other with your hands on a wall. Keeping the back foot facing forward and your heel firmly on the floor, bend your front knee until you feel a stretch in the back of the calf. Hold this stretch for at least 30 seconds. Repeat on the other side.

With your feet in this same position, bend both knees—keeping both heels on the ground—until you feel a stretch a bit lower in the calf. Hold for at least 30 seconds. Repeat one to two times on each side.

Keeping your feet healthy is essential to a vigorous, healthy lifestyle.

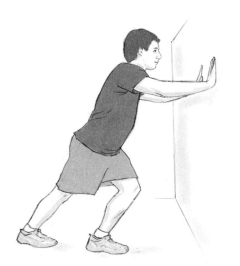
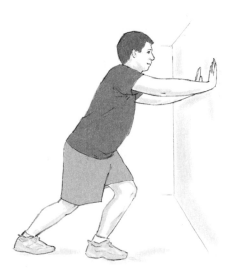

LEARN IT!

- Dopamine, the feel-good chemical that affects the pleasure centers in your brain, lies at the heart of addiction.

- When super-high amounts of dopamine are released on a repeated basis, larger and larger amounts are needed to produce the same effect.

- Genetic alterations in dopamine receptors can predispose one to addiction.

- The gene D2R2 codes for a dopamine receptor that does not readily recognize dopamine. It is found in 50 to 80 percent of those addicted to drugs.

- You can learn to manipulate your own dopamine levels through behavior.

- Smoking is the leading cause of preventable death in the United States.

- Your amygdala cannot activate the stress response when you are eating. This partially explains emotional eating: it temporarily relaxes you.

PERSONALIZE IT!

This week, work on your Motivated Brain.

Your behavior is influenced by a chemical called dopamine. This chemical is released by "pleasure centers" in your brain, and it captures your attention and drives your motivation toward a behavior. Learn to structure your healthy behaviors around simple, healthy things that you enjoy. In this way, you can both promote motivation and structure a lifestyle that is not only healthy but sustainable.

Here are some examples of how people in The Program have personalized this brain principle and put it into action.

- Julie O., a 51-year-old writer, needed motivation to exercise and eat well. She decided to reward herself for meeting her goals by setting up a point system that she could cash in at intervals for a massage or pedicure.

- Lisa N., a 47-year-old mother of two, had a group of friends who walked together every day after the kids went to school. The friends all had children, so the walking was as much a parent support group and social hour as it was an exercise group. The social camaraderie motivated Lisa.

- Steve N., a 51-year-old business owner, had done a lot of sports in the past, and he enjoyed being part of a team. He found motivation to exercise through the organization Team in Training. He enjoyed sharing his exercise time with new and inspiring friends while training for a marathon.

- Connie P., a 35-year-old doctor, found she looked forward to running more if she combined her running with listening to books on tape. Her busy life never allowed time for pleasure reading, so this became her motivation for exercise.

- Joe H., a 62-year-old project manager, had type 2 diabetes. Joe needed to track his blood sugar level more closely. His partner gave him an incentive: if he maintained his blood sugar level below a certain range 75 percent of the time each month, his partner would take him to an art museum or symphony, his two biggest passions. This encouraged him to watch his blood sugar level more carefully while also adding an incentive that made it more fun.

- John and Linda C., both in their forties, decided to do their exercise routine together with their kids, who were 10 and 13 years old. Three nights a week, the family played fun, energetic music from a "workout"

CD their kids had created. They jumped rope, ran up and down the stairs of their house, and did resistance and stretching exercises. After their 30 minutes of exercise, the whole family relaxed and watched a favorite TV show together. John and Linda were motivated to do this by the fun they saw their kids having with them and also by the knowledge that they were helping their kids create healthful habits for life.

LIVE IT!

- Review last week's goals and create this week's short term goals.

- Decide whether there is any substance or behavior addiction for which you need help. Remember, people can get addicted to many different things, not just drugs, alcohol, and tobacco. If you feel you are addicted to something and want to quit, look around for support groups in this area or work with a counselor or other health care professional. Breaking an addiction can, without a doubt, be done, and you can certainly do it; however, efforts are most successful with a supportive social infrastructure.

- List some healthy, dopamine-elevating activities that you can incorporate into your daily routine to keep you happy and motivated to live healthfully.

- Think about whether you ever eat emotionally and list some alternative activites you can do instead.

- Take time this week to note all of the positive benefits you are starting to enjoy from the exercise program you are on. Are you feeling calmer? Are you in a better mood? Do you have more energy? Are you sleeping better? Are you feeling more productive, focused, and attentive?

PREVENTING CANCER

Our greatest glory is not in never falling,
but in rising up every time we fall.

–RALPH WALDO EMERSON

CANCER IS SECOND ONLY to heart disease as the leading cause of death in the United States, but people usually fear cancer more than they fear heart problems. This is understandable. Cancer can be cruel. Although the disease and its treatment can be quite complex, understanding the nature of cancer itself is pretty simple.

It works like this. Every cell in your body has the capacity to replicate, but this ability is controlled by a very tight checks-and-balances system. In cancer, the genes that control this checks-and-balances system become damaged. The proteins produced by these damaged genes are altered in either quality or quantity, and the delicate checks-and-balances system is destroyed. The cell starts to multiply over and over without inhibition, forming a tumor. Eventually some of these cancerous cells slip into the bloodstream and are carried to distant organs of the body such as the liver, brain, or bone, a process known as *metastasis*. There, the cells grow satellite tumors that again are unchecked. It is usually the physical presence of the tumor at either the original or satellite site that creates the symptoms that lead to the diagnosis of cancer. Of course, the earlier you discover the cancer, especially before it has metastasized, the easier it is to cure it. In cancer treatment, *all* cancerous cells must be destroyed. Otherwise, they will continue to replicate unchecked.

What damages a cell's genes in the first place, you ask? Good question. Sometimes people are born with genetic mutations that contribute to the development of cancer. In virtually all cases, however, environmental insults are also required to tip the balance. Food toxins, viruses, air pollutants, ultraviolet radiation—all are examples of environmental insults that can damage a cell's DNA. P53 is a tumor suppressor protein. In 50 percent of cancers a defective P53 protein is found. The P53 protein prevents the cells from replicating recklessly. Unchecked replication can lead to more DNA mistakes, which can then lead to cancer.

The risk of an American man developing cancer over his lifetime is one in two. The leading cancer sites in order of frequency for men are prostate (33%), lung (13%), and colon (10%). Even though prostate cancer is the most frequent cancer in men, lung cancer is by far the most common fatal cancer. Lung cancer accounts for 31 percent of male cancer deaths, followed by colon (10%) and prostate (9%) cancers.

Approximately one in three women in the United States will develop cancer over her lifetime. The leading sites in order of frequency are breast (31%), lung (12%), and colon (11%). In women, lung cancer also causes the highest fatality rates at 26 percent, followed by breast (15%) and colon (10%) cancers.

Although it may feel as if a lot is out of your control, the fact is that you can actually have an enormous impact in reducing your risk of cancer. How? By living healthfully. *It is estimated that 50 percent of cancer is preventable.*

Let's start with tobacco. Although there has been a dramatic fall in the number of smokers in the United States, the smoking frequency today is still 23 percent for men and 19 percent for women. Education correlates inversely with smoking. The more education you have, the less likely you are to smoke. Only 12 percent of college graduates smoke. Here's an interesting bit of information. Did you know that 90 percent of adult smokers started smoking before the age of 18? That means that if a child can make it to his or her 18th birthday without acquiring a smoking habit, there is a good chance that he or she will remain tobacco-free for the rest of his life.

If you smoke, the single most important thing you can do to prevent cancer is to stop. If all you did in The Program was to stop smoking, you would improve your health status tenfold. Smoking accounts for 90 percent of lung cancer, but it also increases the risk of cancer in the mouth, throat, nasal cavities, larynx, esophagus, pancreas, kidney, bladder, cervix, and bone marrow. Chewing tobacco and secondhand smoke cause cancer as well. Smokers who quit can expect to live ten years longer than someone who continues to smoke. I know it isn't easy to stop, but, as I mentioned last week, there is more help now for someone who wants to stop smoking than ever before.

Obesity is the largest nonsmoking lifestyle cause of cancer deaths in the United States. In spite of this, obesity rates continue to rise, especially in children and adolescents. Obesity is a significant risk factor for breast, uterine, kidney, and esophageal cancers and has a moderate effect on colon cancer. How significant a role obesity plays in cancer ranges from 10 to 40 percent depending on the type of cancer. Studies suggest that obesity in the United States may account for 14 percent of cancer deaths in men and 20 percent of cancer deaths in women.

Physical activity reduces your risk of cancer. Men over 65 who exercise regularly have a 70 percent lower risk of developing prostate cancer than their sedentary counterparts. Physically active men and women enjoy a 60 percent decrease in the risk of colon cancer. Regular exercise reduces a woman's risk of breast cancer by 50 percent. Exercise stimulates the production of immune cells that hunt down and destroy cancer cells. Try to get in at least 30 minutes of moderately intense exercise most days of the week to help prevent cancer.

It's clear that having a normal weight and exercising both protect against cancer. What about healthful eating? Studies that evaluate the role of nutrition in the reduction of cancer have produced mixed results. Diets high in saturated and trans fats are thought to increase the risk of some cancers. The recommendation by the American Cancer Society is to eat at least five servings of fruits and vegetables per day, eat whole grains instead of refined grains, and minimize consumption of saturated and trans fats as well as red meat. To date, there have been no studies supporting a clear benefit in cancer reduction by taking vitamin pills or supplements. Recently, low vitamin D levels have been associated with higher overall mortality and a higher risk of certain cancers. Although it is too early to tell if taking more vitamin D will actually reduce cancer, it is currently suggested that those older than 50 take a vitamin D supplement of 800 IU a day.

Limit alcohol consumption to no more than one drink per day for women and two drinks per day for men. More leads to an increase in the frequency of breast, colon, mouth, and esophageal cancers. Alcohol may also promote higher rates of liver cancer in the presence of chronic hepatitis B or C.

Avoid excess sun. Skin cancer is directly related to sun exposure. The ultraviolet radiation damages the DNA of skin cells, increasing the risk of cancerous changes. Don't visit tanning booths; they emit ultraviolet A radiation. Both UVA and UVB increase the risk of cancer. Wear sunscreen with SPF 15 or higher and UVA or UVB protection.

Practice safe sex to reduce the incidence of cancer-promoting viruses such as human immunodeficiency virus (HIV), human papillomavirus (HPV), and hepatitis B and C that spread through blood and body fluid.

Certainly if you live healthfully, you will have a lower probability of developing cancer, but cancer can randomly occur in anyone. As unfair as that is, it can happen. If it does, you want to catch it as early as possible. This is where cancer screening comes in. The purpose of screening is to find cancer in its very early stages. Here are some guidelines for cancer screening.

CANCER PREVENTION GUIDELINES

- **Cervical cancer.** Pap smears should start at age 21 or within three years from the onset of sexual activity, whichever comes first. The recommended frequency for Pap smears is every one to three years. The Pap smear tests for cervical cancer, which is slow-growing and extremely preventable if women follow these guidelines. Pap smears can be discontinued at around age 70 if the previous three Pap smears have been completely normal. The presence of HPV, which can promote the development of cervical cancer, can also be screened for in a Pap smear specimen. The HPV vaccine is now available for cervical cancer prevention and is recommended for all women age 26 and under.

- **Breast cancer.** Mammograms should start at age 40 for most women and are recommended yearly. Baseline mammograms are no longer performed at age 35 because breasts are still so dense at this age that it makes the interpretation of the mammogram too difficult.

- **Colon cancer.** Colonoscopies are recommended for everyone starting at age 50. If the first colonoscopy is negative and there is no family history of colon cancer, screening once every ten years is probably fine. If a precancerous polyp is found during a colonoscopy, screening should be more frequent, usually once every three years until several colonoscopies have been clear; after that, you can extend the screening to once every five years.

  If you have a family history of colon cancer (or precancerous polyps), screening colonoscopies should begin at age 40 and be repeated every five years. Colonoscopies may be recommended earlier if you have a history of family members who have developed colon cancer at a very young age or have certain conditions that accelerate the likelihood of developing colon cancer, such as ulcerative colitis or Crohn's colitis.

- **Prostate cancer** is screened for by a prostate exam (palpation of the prostate by rectal exam) and a blood test called prostate-specific antigen (PSA). Although the guidelines vary, the prostate exam and blood test are typically done in men every year after age 50. Prostate screening may begin earlier in patients with a family history of prostate cancer or those who fall into a higher risk category, such as African Americans.

- **Skin cancer** checks should be done yearly at the time you have your physical exam to check for cancerous or precancerous lesions.

Allen was 57 years old when he started to have rectal bleeding. A colonoscopy showed that he had colon cancer. Unfortunately, he had skipped the screening colonoscopy at age 50, so by the time it was found, the cancer had already spread to a spot in Allen's liver. He underwent resection of his colon as well as removal of the single liver lesion. He underwent chemotherapy and radiation. Later, two other lesions appeared in his lungs, and these were also removed surgically.

Allen's case was atypical. Colon cancer is usually not surgically removed from multiple metastatic areas. Even with these surgeries, however, Allen's blood indicated that he still had colon cancer somewhere in his system, and it seemed as though it would only be a matter of time before the cancer reappeared. Allen continued to be optimistic, though. He did not know what the future held, and he felt there was really nothing he could do but enjoy the present, so he did. He was utterly remarkable in the way he maintained his sense of humor and spirits. One day last year, a couple of years after his last surgery, without any further medical intervention, Allen's blood work came back clear, no longer showing any markers for the presence of cancer. A full year later, Allen remains in remission. His CT scans have remained negative.

I continue to be amazed by this case, mostly because of the attitude Allen demonstrated throughout his treatment. Also, in spite of what he was going through, he never stopped reaching out to help others. He became a leader in several local and national cancer support groups. He never lost his sense of humor and love of life. I do believe his attitude helped strengthen his immune system to rally around his disease.

Ginger was only 30 years old when she discovered a breast lump. Although her young age was unusual for cancer, she was diagnosed with invasive breast cancer and ultimately had to have both breasts surgically removed. She was not married. She had been working nonstop for a start-up company and did not even have a social support network at the time of her treatment. When she went home from the hospital with drains still attached, she was all alone. She had a long and difficult recovery, undergoing both chemotherapy and radiation. Ultimately, the cancer appeared entirely cured, but she had to look at how she would live the rest of her life. She had been working nonstop, and she did not want to keep up the frantic pace. So she decided to make some major life changes. She decided to leave her job.

This of course took guts, but Ginger was incredibly resilient. She somehow managed to pick herself up and keep going. She was even able to see some of the positive things that resulted from her ordeal. She no longer needed success at work to define her. She realized she needed to slow down and enjoy life. She learned to seek social support and started reaching out to others. In addition to seeing a counselor, she became involved in a cancer support group, helping others so that she could give back to her community. Although the experience was one she said she would not wish upon anyone, she felt she emerged from it stronger and better. It is remarkable how resilient human beings can be in extremely difficult situations, and Ginger was able to take a bad situation and emerge stronger, happier, and ultimately healthier.

Although you can't *fully* protect yourself from cancer, there is much you can do to minimize your risk. We are all capable of decreasing our cancer risks by simply adopting a healthier lifestyle.

NUTRITION: PORTION DISTORTION

"Portion distortion" is a catchy phrase that means just what it says. That is, our perception of what constitutes a normal serving size has become distorted over time. It's shocking, but if you look at what food portions were like in this country as recently as the 1950s, you'll see that *portions have doubled in size*. In the 1950s, a bagel weighed two ounces. Now a bagel weighs five to six ounces. A cookie weighed half an ounce. Now most cookies weigh four ounces. A Coca-Cola came in a six-ounce bottle. Now a Coca-Cola comes in a twenty-ounce can. A serving of McDonald's fries weighed two ounces. Now a large serving of McDonald's fries weighs six ounces.

One reason for portion distortion is that food industries are simply packaging much greater quantities of food and charging roughly the same price. Food has become cheap and abundant. Because of advances in technology, food production has become almost too efficient. *The United States now produces twice as much food as it needs to feed its population.* Food industries deal with this excess food by packaging a larger volume of food and selling it for a price that is only marginally higher than the price of a smaller size. Just look at the price difference between a small and a medium bag of popcorn the next time you go to the movies. Americans like a bargain and see no reason not to purchase the larger size if they see it as a better value. The danger in this, though, is that the more you give people to eat, the more they tend to eat.

This "see food, eat it" phenomenon is well documented. It has been observed in a variety of studies in all age groups. In one study, moviegoers were randomly given a medium or large container of free popcorn that was either fresh or stale. Those eating from the larger container of fresh popcorn ate 45 percent more than those who received a medium container of popcorn. And even though the people who had the stale popcorn didn't really like it, they still ate 34 percent more when it was served in a large container instead of a medium container. In a recent study, young children ate more when they were served more food. It has long been thought that young children had good self-regulation of appetite and would eat only until satisfied. Several recent studies fail to support this.

As mentioned before, it makes sense from an evolutionary standpoint that we would have evolved the tendency to want to eat all food in front of us. A million years ago, starvation was not a rare cause of death. Our evolutionary ancestors never knew when their next calorie was coming. But we aren't living on the savanna, hunting and gathering, anymore, so this biologic wiring now works against us.

This trend toward larger portions has been big news over the last several years. The popular documentary *Super Size Me* drew attention to the problem. After the movie came out, McDonald's did away with its supersize options, but for the most part, the megaportions in the food industry have continued. One fast-food chain on the East Coast recently created the Monster Thickburger, with more than 1,400 calories.

The sad fact is that we are becoming a nation of Mega-Americans. The national weight gain of the average American over the last fifty years is no secret, and it is no small matter. The dramatic rise in the number of Americans considered overweight or obese has catapulted obesity into the national health spotlight; it is now considered one of the highest national health priorities.

As you know by now, the concern over weight has nothing to do with cosmetics. Obesity is second only to smoking as a predictor of health problems and health care costs. Obesity contributes to diabetes, hypertension, elevated cholesterol, heart disease, cancer, arthritis, sleep apnea, and esophageal reflux. Today, two thirds of the people in our country are classified as overweight or obese.

Portion distortion is not the only reason our nation has become so obese. We live in a time when technology has largely relieved us of the need to move. The food choices that are convenient and ever present tend to be high in calories and low in nutritional content. But because they are convenient, they have become a staple in our diet. We are also a nation that moves so fast and tries to accomplish

OBESITY DENSITIES IN THE U.S.

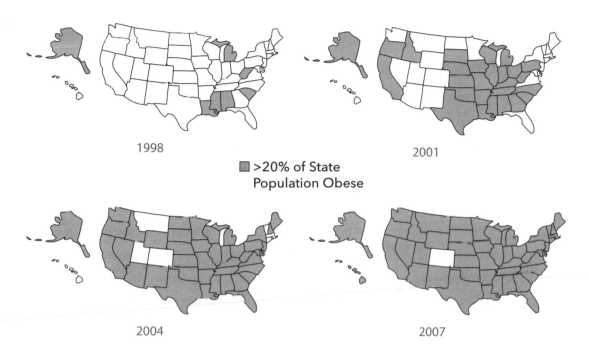

1998

2001

■ >20% of State
Population Obese

2004

2007

so much that high stress levels are now the norm for many people. Stress is not good for health in the first place, but it also contributes to weight gain when food is used to relax and comfort. With such busy lives, people also tend to cut back on the amount of sleep they get, and, as we saw in Week 7, this can contribute to weight gain as well.

This week, pay particular attention to your portions. Portion control is fundamental to eating healthfully and maintaining an ideal body weight, both of which are so important to your overall health. Here are some tips to help you keep your portion sizes reasonable.

- **Use smaller plates when you serve yourself food.** You may think that this is way too simplistic and that your brain cannot be fooled so easily, but it actually works. Try using ten-inch plates instead of twelve-inch plates at lunch and dinner. If you have a small plate that is filled, you are more likely to feel full after a meal than if you have a large plate that was only half full with the same amount of food. Try it, it works!

- **Practice taking the same amount of food you normally eat at a meal and cutting it in half.** You can still eat the rest, but wait twenty minutes to see whether you are still hungry. It takes twenty minutes for the body to release chemicals that tell your brain you are satisfied. Most people eat their meals in less than twenty minutes, so they end up eating more than they really need to. The point of this exercise is to show you that it takes far less food to satisfy your hunger than you may think.

- **Start leaving a little of every meal behind on your plate** and make it a habit of throwing it into the garbage immediately after you have finished eating. You need to get used to not feeling that you should eat absolutely everything you have on your plate.

- **Keep the serving plates in the kitchen instead of on the dinner table;** otherwise, the visual cue of the food on the table can encourage overeating.

- It is always a good idea to intermittently break out measuring cups and spoons and **practice measuring your food portions**. Compare measured food servings to your fist to estimate one cup or to your palm to estimate a half cup or a three-ounce standard portion of meat. Even though you have done this before, it is good to remind yourself from time to time.

- **Get into the habit of brushing your teeth right after a meal** so you aren't tempted to keep eating.

- **Try chewing a stick of gum or have a breath mint or breath strip mint after a meal.** These techniques overwhelm the taste buds and often extinguish postmeal sweet cravings.

- **Practice turning off the lights in the kitchen after dinner and saying out loud, "I have finished eating for the day."** This last strategy might seem silly and it may amuse your kids, spouse, or roommate, but it works.

GERD

Large food portions increase the risk of developing gastroesophageal reflux disease (GERD), which occurs when the acidic stomach contents pass back up into the esophagus. This happens when the pressure in the stomach exceeds the pressure exerted by the lower esophageal sphincter muscle. Once stomach acid reaches the esophagus, there is little to stop it from traveling to your throat, sinuses, larynx, or lungs, especially after meals and at night when you are lying flat. Common signs and symptoms of GERD may include heartburn, regurgitation, sore throat, halitosis (bad breath), throat clearing, globus (sensation of fullness in the throat), hoarseness, sinusitis, chronic cough, asthma, sleep apnea, and in a small number of cases even laryngeal cancer and esophageal cancer. Forty percent of the U.S. population will have acute or chronic GERD at some point in their lives. Like most diseases, whether or not you develop GERD is a function of your genetics to some extent and of lifestyle to a much larger extent. Here are the things you can do to minimize the risk of GERD.

1 **Do not lie down within three hours of eating,** as your stomach is still full. It takes three hours for your stomach to empty.

2 **Do not lie down within two hours of drinking liquids,** even water. Keep hydrated during the day, but don't drink right before you go to bed.

3 **Eat small, frequent meals** so your stomach remains under less pressure.

4 **Try to avoid things that relax the esophageal sphincter** and keep it from doing its job. Such things include cigarette smoking, alcohol, caffeine, chocolate, and fats.

5 **See your doctor if you have continued symptoms of GERD** despite
these lifestyle changes, as this condition is usually progressive but can
be treated successfully.

People practice portion control in all sorts of different ways. Phil, a 39-year-old farmer from Beaver Dam, Ohio, found that he did better if his wife put the food on his plate and kept all the food platters in the kitchen. This helped him stay away from seconds. Judy, a 51-year-old mom from Seattle, decided to buy snack foods already divided into little packages rather than eating from big containers. She liked to shop at Costco, though, so when she bought things in big containers, she found it worked just as well to make up her own snack packages. Sally, a 72-year-old retired teacher from Birmingham, Michigan, found that she ate a lot more when she was around other people who ate a lot. Just realizing this helped her become more aware and curb her portions.

FITNESS: PROTECTING AND STRENGTHENING YOUR JOINTS

Ankles

Ankle injuries are common. An ankle sprain can leave your ankle vulnerable to future sprains because the damaged nerve fibers around the ankle are no longer able to sense the ankle's exact position. Fortunately, there are strengthening exercises that can prevent future sprains by rehabilitating these nerve fibers and strengthening the muscles that support the ankle. You can also do these exercises to prevent an ankle sprain from happening in the first place.

The first exercise strengthens the inside and outside of the ankle—very important for lateral (sideways) movement. Sit in a chair in a room with a hard-surfaced floor (linoleum, hardwood, or tile). Place a bath towel on the floor with one end of it under the ball of your right foot. Keeping your knee still and your heel on the floor, push the towel away from the rest of it by sliding it over, picking up the ball of your foot, and sliding it again. Do this movement repeatedly until you reach the other end of the towel, or until your ankle feels fatigued. Once you get to the end, slide the towel in the opposite direction. If you keep your knee still and your heel in contact with the floor, you will be working the exact muscles that support your ankle against a sprain. Perform 2 to 3 repetitions in each direction. Repeat on the other side.

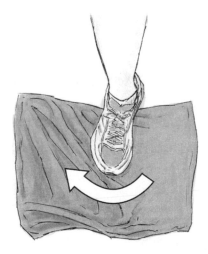

Next, practice balancing on one foot. You should be able to balance on one foot for 2 minutes without losing your balance. To work on this, stand next to a wall or other sturdy object that you can reach if you need to. Keeping your standing leg slightly bent and your hip, knee, and ankle in alignment, hold this position for up to 2 minutes before switching to the other side.

If you'd like to challenge yourself more, start in the same position as in the previous exercise, but add a toe raise. When you rise up onto your toes, imagine a straight line from your hip, knee, and ankle through your second toe (the one next to your big toe). Slowly rise up and then lower yourself while balancing. Repeat 10 to 15 times, then switch to the other side.

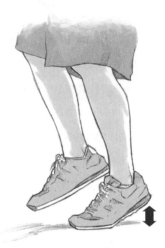

Many foot and ankle injuries are caused by worn-out shoes or the classic "too much, too soon" scenario. If you are starting a new exercise program, remember to begin slowly and increase no more than 10 percent each week. Exercise shoes should be sports-specific (for example, court shoes for tennis and basketball, running shoes for jogging and walking). Most important, *shoes need to be replaced regularly.* If you are exercising three to five days per week, you should replace your shoes about every six months to prevent injuries. Lower-extremity injuries heal slowly because your lower extremities are in constant use, so icing is necessary to decrease inflammation and pain. Non-weight-bearing exercise (swimming, pool jogging, biking) will also speed the recovery of foot and ankle injuries. If you follow these guidelines, you can go a long way toward keeping your ankles strong and preventing future injuries.

Forearms

We use our forearms all day long. The muscles that control the movement of your wrist and fingers originate at the elbow and travel through the forearm into the wrist, hand, and fingers. Whether you are typing, using your computer mouse, driving a car, writing, lifting, or doing any other activity with your arms, you are utilizing very small muscles repeatedly—so much so that you can easily overuse these muscles and cause dysfunction and pain. Even the simple motion of turning a key in a door can aggravate an already overused forearm.

When you use your forearm muscles, they are repeatedly contracted and shortened. This fact makes it all the more important that you stretch them frequently. Think of the "front" of your forearm as that on the same side as the palm of your hand. To stretch the front of your forearm, place your arm straight out in front of you with your palm up. Use your opposite hand to press your fingers and hand toward the floor until you feel a stretch in the front of your forearm. Hold this stretch for 30 seconds.

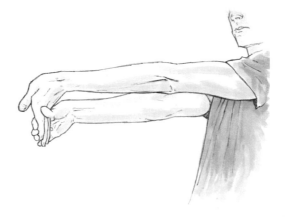

The other side of your forearm also needs to be stretched. To do this, you need to make a gentle fist with your arm out in front of you. Keeping your arm in front of you, direct your fist toward the ground, then rotate it down and away from your midline until you feel a stretch along the (now) top of your forearm. If you need to, you can use your opposite hand to provide gentle overpressure. Hold this stretch for 30 seconds. Perform both of these stretches on each side several times a day, especially if you use your hands a lot.

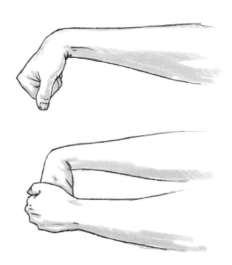

One way to keep your forearm muscles in shape for their high level of activity is to strengthen them appropriately. Because these are small muscles that are used a lot, you need to train them that way—use light resistance with a high number of repetitions in a set. A light resistance band works just fine. Rest your forearm on a sturdy surface, with your elbow close to your side. Make a loop with your band and step on one end of it. Hold the band with your hand palm down. Keep your forearm still and pull the band up toward the ceiling. Slowly return to the start position. Perform 20 to 30 repetitions. Repeat on the other side.

In order to work the "front" of the forearm, start in the same position as before, but with your palm facing the ceiling. Lift just your hand toward the ceiling, keeping your forearm still. Return to the start position and repeat 20 to 30 times. Repeat on the other side.

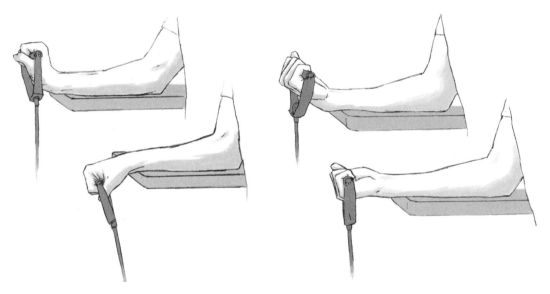

Even if you stretch and strengthen your forearms consistently, it is still possible to aggravate these muscles with everyday activities such as computer use. If you are on a computer for most of the day, there are some things you can try. Consider training yourself to use your mouse on your nondominant side. This minimizes the stress of your dominant side's forearm—which is being used for typing, number keying, writing, and so on. Also, don't "plant" and "pivot" the heel of your hand on a pad when you are keyboarding or using your mouse. This places excessive strain on the carpal tunnel, a cluster of bones in your wrist through which a nerve passes through to the fingers.

No matter what activities you do throughout the day, make sure your posture is appropriate for the task. Keep your ears over your shoulders and your shoulders over your hips. Whether you are sitting or standing, it is ideal to keep your elbows as close to your body as possible to avoid excessive strain on the neck and arms.

Once you have established good posture, be vigilant about taking frequent breaks. Just standing up and sitting back down to "reset" your sitting position can help you avoid overuse issues in your entire upper body. Keep all of this in mind throughout each day, and you can minimize the stress on your wrist/elbow complex.

Knees

Your knees are responsible for keeping you mobile, getting you out of a chair or car, and allowing you to climb and descend different terrains. It is important to protect them as much as possible. Avoid fully squatting repeatedly and pressing your knees into a hyperextended position. Repeated twisting over your knees can also create problems, as can stressing your knees with high intensity impact over long periods of time. The name of the game is to keep the muscles around your knees strong. This is the very best way to protect your knee joints.

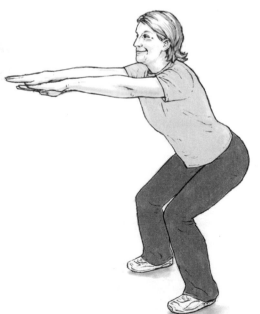

There are three easy exercises you can do to strengthen the knees. Two of these three are included in the resistance exercises introduced in Week 5. The first exercise is the Squat. Stand with your feet shoulder width apart. Bend your knees and keep your weight on your heels so your knees do not protrude past your toes. Keep your chest lifted, and don't let your knees drift inward toward each other during the movement.

Bend to achieve just above a ninety-degree angle in your knees and then slowly stand back up. Repeat 10 to 15 times.

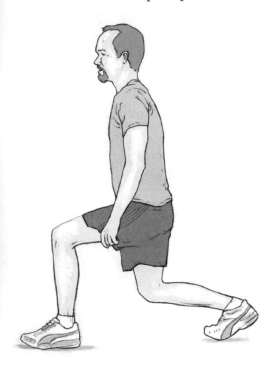

The second exercise is the Modified Lunge. Stand with your feet in a "stride-step" position. Lower your back knee while lifting that heel off of the floor. Lower until your front knee is just above a ninety-degree angle. Don't let your knees protrude past your toes, and keep your chest lifted. Slowly return to the start position. Repeat this 10 to 15 times, then switch sides. This exercise also challenges your balance—an added bonus!

The third and final exercise is called the Bridge. This exercise strengthens the hamstrings and calves and stretches the quadriceps, all at the same time. Lie on your back with your knees bent and your feet flat on the floor. Keeping your abdomen pulled in, lift your buttocks off the floor until your knees, hips, and shoulders create a straight line. Slowly lower back to the start position. Repeat 10 to 15 times. If this seems pretty easy, do the exact same exercise, but start with one foot off of the ground and lift with the other, keeping your hips level and even. These simple exercises will go a long way toward keeping your knees healthy.

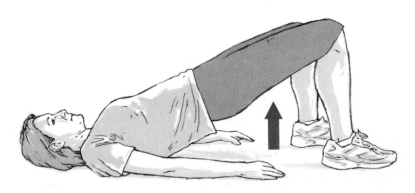

Lower Back

Lower-back pain is the most common reason people go to a doctor's office. It may be something that happens suddenly, but most often it is a chronic problem that comes and goes sporadically. Generally speaking, the more healthfully you live, the less likely you are to have lower-back pain. Being fit definitely helps to decrease back pain and helps to keep it from happening in the first place.

Proper posture is important in managing lower-back pain. More specifically, finding the neutral position of your spine is the key. The neutral spine is the position in which your lower back feels most comfortable. It is the position in the middle of an arched back and a rounded back. This position is different for each person, and it depends on your anatomy as well as your history of back pain.

To find your neutral spine, lie on your back with your knees bent and your feet flat on the floor. If you are comfortable in this position and have no back pain, this is probably your neutral spine.

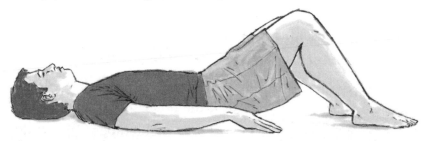

If you still are not comfortable, slightly arch or round your lower back until you feel pain-free and comfortable. This arching and rounding is done by performing the Pelvic Tilt. You can tilt your pelvis backward by pulling your belly button toward your spine and squeezing your buttocks. Together, these two muscle groups control the position of your pelvis. The more you contract them, the more your lower back rounds and flattens toward the floor. By relaxing these muscles, your lower back will relax and naturally return to a slightly arched position.

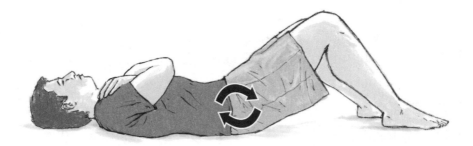

The point of the Pelvic Tilt is to move your pelvis until your lower back is in a neutral position and then to hold that position. Once you are able to find your neutral spine, you want to be able to use the lower abdominal and buttocks muscles to hold you in this position.

You've probably heard how important your "core" is, right? Your core muscles are those that maintain and support your neutral spine. You can essentially work your core just by holding your spine in a neutral position while you do any other activity or exercise.

For example, while holding your back in a neutral spine position, slowly lift one foot just a few inches off the floor. Don't let your pelvis rock or your lower back rise out of position. Then slowly place that foot back on the floor before you lift the opposite foot. Pay close attention to how your pelvis automatically shifts when you place one foot down and pick the other up. Your mission is to avoid *any* movement through your hips and pelvis by tightening your core and buttocks muscles. Imagine a glass of water balancing on your abdomen. Don't let it tip over!! Repeat this exercise 10 to 15 times on each side.

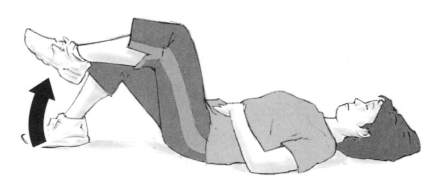

You can also challenge your core by finding your neutral spine in a different position. Get down on your hands and knees. Arch and round your lower back by doing the Pelvic Tilt until you find your neutral spine—your back should be relatively flat from your shoulders to your hips (and this position should be pain-free). Once you've found your neutral spine, lift your right arm forward and up, so it is in line with your body. But don't move out of your neutral spine position! Whenever your arms go above your head, your lower back will have a tendency to arch and therefore move out of the neutral position. In order to avoid this, you need to do the Pelvic Tilt just enough to prevent your lower back from arching. The higher you reach, the more you need to do the Pelvic Tilt to maintain the neutral position. Hold the arm up for a few seconds, then lower it back to the floor. Alternate arms and repeat 10 to 15 times on each side.

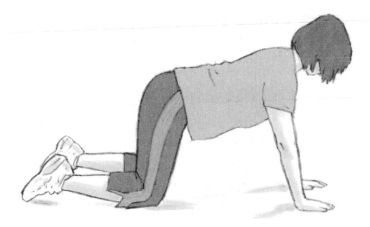

For a slightly harder challenge, instead of lifting your arm, lift one leg straight out behind you. Remember, the most important part of this exercise is holding your lower back in the neutral spine position. If you are unable to maintain this position when you lift your arm or leg, the entire exercise loses its purpose. Hold your leg out for a few seconds, then lower it back to the floor. Alternate legs and repeat 10 to 15 times on each side. Remember that imaginary glass of water on your tummy? Now imagine it balancing on the small of your back—don't let it tip when you are switching sides.

If you really want to challenge yourself, put the two exercises together: lift the opposite arm and leg at the same time while maintaining the neutral spine. This exercise not only works your core and reinforces the neutral spine position, it is also a great exercise for balance! So the neutral spine is your position of comfort. You contract your abdominal muscles by pulling your tummy away from your waist and squeezing your buttocks muscles to tilt your pelvis into a neutral position. Once you are in neutral, these same muscle groups are responsible for holding the position. If you can maintain the neutral spine while performing everyday activities and/or exercising, you will be able to protect your lower back from undue stress. This is an easy concept but difficult in practice.

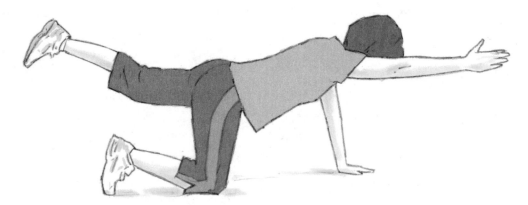

Performing the exercises we've talked about is just the beginning of mastering this concept. There are also other ways to protect your back: do not lift, twist, or bend with your lower back; if you are lifting an object, lift with your legs and carry it close to your body; and avoid staying in one position for long periods of time. If you are vigilant with all of this, I am confident that you will be able to manage your lower-back pain or prevent it from occuring altogether.

Poor posture is the most common cause of neck pain. We often sit, stand, and work in awkward positions that contribute to neck strain. Whether you are sitting or standing, try to remember to keep your ears, shoulders, and hips in line with one another. This will facilitate better posture and limit stress and strain on your neck.

One exercise that can strengthen postural muscles is the Shoulder Blade Squeeze. Sit or stand with your hips, shoulders, and ears in alignment and your arms at your sides. Without arching your lower back, turn your palms forward, then out while squeezing your shoulder blades together. Make sure your shoulders don't shrug during this movement. Hold your shoulder blades together for two to three seconds, then relax. Repeat 5 times. Since this exercise can be done anywhere, practice it several times a day. It will help you keep your posture "up to par" throughout the day.

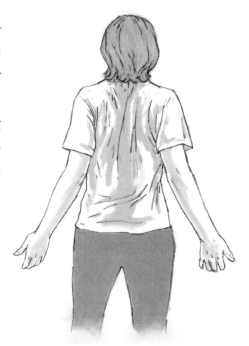

There are small but important muscles in your neck that are often overstretched and weakened over time with poor posture. These are the deep neck flexors, and they help to keep your head in a good position over your neck. Weakness in these muscles contributes to neck and headache pain. To strengthen them, you can do Chin Nods. Sit or stand in good alignment. Next, bring the bottom of your chin toward your Adam's apple, hold for two to three seconds, and then relax. The motion should create a bit of a double chin. Repeat 5 times. Just like the Shoulder Blade Squeeze, this exercise can be done several times during the day and will help maintain good posture.

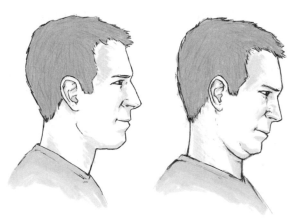

Remember, when it comes to your neck, proper posture is the most important thing. Keep your ears over your shoulders and your shoulders over your hips. Be aware of your posture at all times. Don't hold the phone with your shoulder, and position your car seat so your entire spine is aligned. Any position held for a long time will eventually create bad posture, so make sure to change your position often (every 20 to 30 minutes or so) or take a break from your position by doing the exercises that we talked about. And do your neck exercises. A strong neck is a healthy, happy neck.

Shoulders

The shoulder joint is complex because of its large range of motion and the mixture of large and small muscles that surround it. The key to a healthy shoulder is balancing range of motion with the strength of these muscles. Common causes of shoulder pain are tendonitis and bursitis. These conditions occur less often when the muscles surrounding the shoulder are strong.

To maintain a good range of motion, perform the next three movements a few times a week.

1 Clasp your hands overhead, then lower them behind your head. Next, pull your elbows as far back as you comfortably can. Hold for 10 seconds.

2 Hold your hands behind you. Slowly slide your hands up your back as far as you comfortably can and hold for 10 seconds.

3 Give yourself a hug—literally. Reach around the backs of your shoulders with both hands as far as you comfortably can. Hold for 10 seconds.

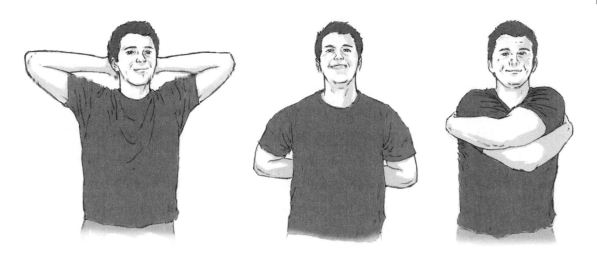

We often live and work with our shoulders rolled forward, so it is important to learn how to strengthen your upper-back muscles. This will help keep the shoulders in a safe position as well as maintain good posture. A great exercise for the upper-back muscles is the Row. Place a resistance band around a sturdy object at chest height, or close the knotted middle of the band in a door. Hold the ends of the band and walk backward away from the door until the band is taut, with your arms straight out in front of you. Begin the exercise by pulling your elbows behind you and squeezing your shoulder blades together. Slowly return to the start position. Repeat 10 to 15 times.

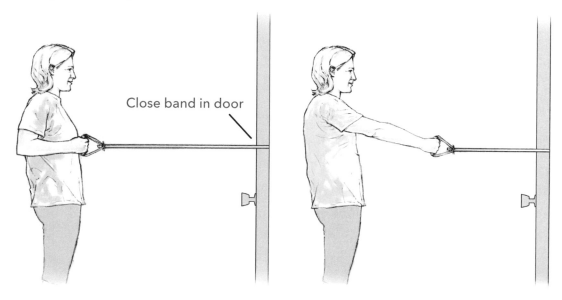

Close band in door

The smaller muscles in your shoulder, the rotator cuff muscles, are responsible for holding the "ball" in the "socket" throughout every movement you ask your shoulder to make. The exercises that strengthen these muscles are called Internal and External Rotation, and they require the use of a very light resistance band. First, attach the band to something sturdy or close it in a door at elbow height. For Internal Rotation, grab the end of the band with your right hand, bend your elbow to a ninety-degree angle, and step away from the door until the band is taut (the band is on your right side). Keeping your elbow at your side, rotate your forearm in to your abdomen, and then slowly return to the start position. The resistance should be light enough to be able to perform 20 to 30 repetitions. Repeat on the other side.

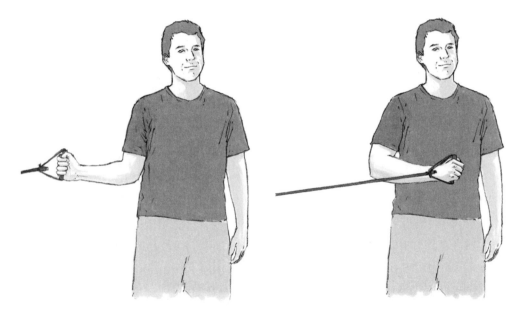

External Rotation is the same movement in the opposite direction (the band is now on your left side). Start with your right hand holding the end of the band, your forearm against your tummy, and then rotate it away, keeping your elbow at your side throughout the entire motion. Again, the resistance should be light enough to do 20 to 30 repetitions. Repeat on the other side.

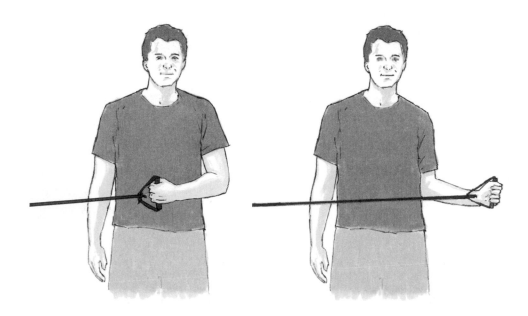

In order to keep your shoulders healthy, you need to maintain both motion and strength. So keep moving your shoulder in all directions and strengthen both the big and small muscles around the joint by doing these exercises at least three times a week. It is important to avoid any pain with these exercises, as working through pain can create secondary dysfunction in the shoulder complex. Strengthen and use your shoulders cautiously and wisely!

LEARN IT!

- It is estimated that 50 percent of cancer is preventable.

- If you smoke, stop. That's the best cancer prevention of all.

- No single vitamin has been shown to prevent cancer.

- The American Cancer Society hotline number is 1-877-937-7848.

- Portion sizes in the United States have doubled since 1950. Pay close attention to portion size, and cut portions in half when you can.

- Two thirds of the U.S. population is classified as overweight or obese. Portion distortion is a major cause of this.

- Joint pain can be prevented or reduced by strengthening the muscles around the joint.

PERSONALIZE IT!

This week, work on your Responsive Brain.

Your health is not predestined by your genes, because your environment turns genes on and off. Your brain responds profoundly to its surrounding environment. When you learn how to optimize your environment, you learn how to turn genes on or off, and for many genes, this translates into behavior. It is crucial to set up your world so that it encourages healthy living.

Here are some examples of how people in The Program have personalized this brain principle and put it into action.

- Kimberley Y., a 41-year-old, found that much of her overeating came from her social life. She went out to eat a lot with friends. She decided to change this so she was not always in front of food. She changed her social get-togethers to revolve around exercise; she invited her friends to go hiking, work out at the gym, and take yoga and Pilates classes together.

- Wendy W., a 32-year-old homemaker, had to ask her husband to stop bringing leftover treats home from his work parties because it was just too tempting to have treats around the house all the time. In fact, she had him take all of *their* leftover treats to his office to share with his work colleagues. She cleared the house of treats quickly after birthday or holiday parties. After Halloween, for example, all leftover candy was immediately sent off to her husband's office. Creating a more healthful environment at home made it easier to maintain good eating habits.

- Peter S., a 35-year-old executive, created fitness competitions at work with colleagues to keep him inspired. For example, in one competition, those who consistently exercised four times a week on average for three months were the winners and were treated to lunch by those who had not met the quota. His efforts helped create a more healthful environment at work, which helped him stay in shape.

- Paula B., 54 years old, found that she was far more inclined to go for a power walk if she laid out her workout clothes before she went to bed so she would be sure to see them first thing in the morning.

LIVE IT!

- Review last week's goals and create this week's short-term goals.

- Check to see that you are up to date on all cancer-screening recommendations, and if not, schedule appointments to get on track.

- Limit sun exposure and wear sunscreen.

- Focus on portions this week.

- If you have a particular joint that bothers you, consider adding some joint-specific exercises to your regimen.

SECRETS OF SUCCESSFUL AGING

In the end, it's not the years in your life that count but the life in your years.

—ABRAHAM LINCOLN

IN THE LAST TEN YEARS, more research has been done on the subject of aging than ever before. Hundreds of studies have looked at whether lifestyle or genetics plays the more important role in the aging process. The good news is that although genes are important in aging, they account for only 20 to 30 percent of how we age. Lifestyle accounts for the rest. What this means is that you are in the driver's seat when it comes to how long and, most important, how well you will live out your later years.

How long is the human life span? The general consensus is that the maximum human life span is about 120 years. In the United States, the current average life span is seventy-eight (for women, eighty years, and for men, seventy-five years). In the United States, despite the fact that the average spending (per person) on health care is grossly higher than any other developed nation, the American life span is a year or two shorter than in other developed countries. This is thought to be largely related to lifestyle issues.

In the past, humans did not reach this maximum human life span because of acute events such as trauma and infection. In the last hundred years, though, amazing strides in medical technology and public health have greatly reduced the death rates from such events. The major cause of early death in humans is now more often from self-inflicted suboptimal lifestyle behaviors. That is, we do too little exercise, eat too much, sleep too little, and stress too much.

Let's review a little of the science behind aging. Why can't we live forever? And how exactly does lifestyle affect the aging process? It all goes back to the cell, the basic unit of life. Each cell's DNA is strung together in the chromosomes, which sit in the command-and-control center of the cell. On the tips of each of these chromosomes are protective caps, called *telomeres,* and with each replication of the chromosome the cap wears down. Once the cap has completely worn down, the chromosome frazzles and clumps, and then the cell dies. Some things speed up this process, and others slow it down. For example, chronic stress shortens the telomere caps. Obesity does, too, probably due to the many inflammatory chemicals secreted by fat cells. Exercise, however, rebuilds the telomeres. Imagine that! Yet another benefit of exercise!

Your body expects this wear and tear; it is designed to withstand some of it. For example, your cell is exposed to a thousand oxidative hits a day. Your body, however, has a built-in repair team that goes around 24/7 repairing the damage. Unfortunately, if your lifestyle involves too much wear and tear on your body, your repair crew will become overwhelmed and unable to keep up.

The three best things you can do to live long and well are: (1) eat a healthy diet, (2) maintain a normal body weight, and (3) do at least 30 minutes of moderately intense exercise most days of the week. That's no surprise: you know that an unhealthy diet, obesity, and a sedentary lifestyle all promote inflammation, which contributes to the relentless wear and tear within each cell.

It should also come as no surprise that part of the formula for living long and well has to do with getting plenty of good-quality sleep, managing daily stress, and avoiding tobacco, excess alcohol, and recreational drugs. Stress and sleep deprivation both increase inflammation. Smoking greatly enhances inflammation and dramatically accelerates aging.

Now let me tell you something you may not know about aging.

Memory

A lot of people worry about their brain function with aging. People often say, "I don't want to live too long—I don't want to stay alive without my brain." Dementia is *not* an inevitable part of aging. In fact, all through life, your brain can continue to develop new pathways and connections between neurons. *Your brain can even make new neurons.* As a person ages, the processing in the brain does slow down, and it does get harder to make those new connections. But you can. That's the important point. And exercise actually helps memory! With exercise, you make higher levels of brain-derived growth factor (BDNF), which enable more connections between the nerve cells and allows new neurons to form. Of course, you have to tell the brain where to make these new connections, and that's why you need to engage in mentally stimulating activities your whole life. It's important to challenge your brain in all sorts of different ways as you get older, so that you stay mentally stimulated and connected to the world around you.

As I've said before, when you exercise, you release growth factors from your muscles, and they go to the brain and provide the infrastructure to lay down new nerve networks. With exercise, you also produce BDNF, which stimulates new nerve production (neurogenesis) and helps you stretch and grow the neurons you already have. If you sprinkle BDNF on a Petri dish of nerve cells, those nerve cells will thrive and grow, sprouting new dendrites like new branches on a young tree in springtime. Here's the key, though: you can exercise all day and have all sorts of growth factors and raw materials ready to go and reshape your brain, but your brain must tell them where to be built. That's where learning comes in. You have to mentally challenge and stimulate your brain so that the new nerve cells know where to go and plug in. When a new nerve cell is born in your brain, it has twenty-eight days to plug into the network or it dies. Learning allows you to insert this new neuron into the network to make good use of it.

In fact, both learning and exercise are critical to warding off Alzheimer's dementia. This disease involves inflammation, so everything we have discussed so far that fights inflammation and keeps your good-guy immune system strong holds true for this disease.

In Alzheimer's disease, a protein called beta-amyloid is deposited on the cable networks of the brain. These deposits gum up the networks so information cannot pass through easily. You do have a protein, APOE4, whose job it is to clean up this mess, but if your lifestyle promotes inflammation, this cleanup process will fall behind. An anti-inflammatory lifestyle therefore helps. Also, mental stimulation promotes the creation of new nerve networks so electrical nerve activity can bypass the gummed-up routes.

In a study in Finland that followed 1,500 Finnish people for twenty-one years, those who exercised at least twice a week were 50 percent less likely to develop dementia than those who didn't. Another study was done on 3,000 nuns, and those who engaged in exercise, learning, and social service were far less likely to develop Alzheimer's than the others. In those who did develop Alzheimer's, the majority of them had not been active mentally or physically when *younger.* So keeping your mind and body active is important throughout your life, not just in the later years. This study was also heartening in that although 37 percent of the nuns showed the pathology of Alzheimer's disease on autopsy, many of those who had been active physically and mentally never showing clinical signs of it in their daily lives. One nun had 90 percent of her brain covered with beta-amyloid, yet she had not demonstrated any memory loss. She had created so many new nerve tracts that bypassed the diseased ones that she had been able to compensate without showing any outward signs of the disease.

In natural aging, there is some slowdown of mental processing. It becomes a little more difficult to retrieve information (such as names and faces) and harder to concentrate and multitask when there are distractions, but learning is always possible.

If you find that your memory is failing you a bit, try these proven memory-enhancing tricks, which work for people at any age.

- **Be selective about what you want to remember.** There are usually only a few major points in any discussion, so try to define what they are.

- **Try saying the points out loud.** Write them down. Read them. Say them out loud again.

- **Work in a place where you can minimize distractions.**

- **Draw key facts out in a diagram or a story.** This gives the brain a different way of storing and later retrieving the information.

- **Ask yourself questions about the information you want to learn.**

- **Use flash cards to force yourself to recall the information.** Your brain remembers things better when you ask it questions or require it to give answers.

- **Make associations of things that are familiar to you with the things you are working to remember.** For example, if you meet someone and her name is Betty, you can make some mental note about her that has to do with your favorite Aunt Betty.

- **Keep all papers organized for easy retrieval.** Maintain a filing system. Have a day planner where you record all your appointments. Have specific places where you keep things such as your keys or glasses.

- **Purge all unnecessary papers and things.** Avoid being a pack rat. It is easier to keep your brain uncluttered if the world around you is organized.

- **Create rituals and mental cues to help you retrieve information.** It is easier to remember to feed the dog or take out the trash if you tie these routines together rather than doing them haphazardly throughout the day.

- **Finally, keep your brain active.** It's just like a muscle in that it needs to be exercised or it atrophies. Use it or lose. Learn a foreign language, play bridge or chess, learn to play a musical instrument, take on new art projects such as watercoloring or sculpturing. Take classes in something you've always been interested in. Force yourself to do new things even if they are a bit out of your comfort zone. In fact, try to push yourself out of your comfort zone on a regular basis. This is how you stimulate your brain to grow. If you are an accountant and your brain is used largely to process numbers, force yourself to take on a more artistic hobby to stretch your brain a little.

Sleep matters in memory because that is when your brain replays what you just learned over and over so that it can make tight connections. Get adequate sleep.

Stress management is important for memory. Stress inhibits both your ability to form new memories and your recall of old memories; it is also toxic to your hippocampus, the memory center.

Mood is important. When a person is depressed, his or her memory is affected until the mood is normalized. You can improve your mood with exercise, counseling, and medication when indicated.

Nutrition is also important for the brain. Your brain depends completely on glucose for its fuel because it does not have the ability to break down fat or protein. It goes through a lot of glucose when you are concentrating hard. So don't skip meals. In fact, it's best for your brain when you eat small, frequent meals. Keep your blood sugar level even by eating whole grains, fruits, vegetables, and lean proteins. Omega-3 fatty acids, found in fatty fish such as salmon, as well as in walnuts, flaxseed, and canola oil, are also thought to have some benefit to the brain, perhaps because of their anti-inflammatory effect.

For optimal aging, in general, establish a relationship with a doctor you trust, and check in on a regular basis to monitor your blood pressure, blood sugar, and cholesterol. You want to make sure your arteries stay clean so that your organs can continue to work well. During your yearly visits, you should also arrange for cancer screening and other preventive checkups.

Another key to healthy aging is attitude. Optimists age better than pessimists. That's a fact. Also, it is important to remain socially connected and involved in at least one activity that lets you feel vital and purposeful. We are social animals; we need to be part of a social network. Studies show that once a person stops feeling that he has a purposeful role in the world outside of himself, he starts to decline. Love, social connection, and laughing all enhance the immune cells and help keep the inflammatory process in check. Studies also show that even if elderly people are fairly isolated socially, if they have a pet (or even plants), their immune system is enhanced and their life span is increased! Sexual arousal also enhances your immune system, so it's not just fun but healthy to keep up your sex life as you age.

What else happens during the aging process? As we age, the levels of many of our hormones start to decline. Growth hormone, which is high in our early years, declines as we age. This hormone promotes growth in our early years and could help repair the wear and tear on our bodies when we are no longer growing. Lots of research has been done on growth hormone to see whether supplementing it helps in the aging process. Unfortunately, these studies have not demonstrated a benefit. Growth hormone may help promote lean muscle, but the side effects of replacement include an increased risk of diabetes, carpal tunnel syndrome, and achy joints, to name just a few.

Dihydroepiandrosterone (DHEA) also declines with age. DHEA is produced by the adrenal glands and is the precursor of testosterone and estrogen. DHEA replacement in the form of a pill has also been evaluated as a possible key to the fountain of youth, but it, too, has failed to show proven benefit when given as a supplement. Exercise though, does drive the natural production of both growth hormone and DHEA. Oh, did I bring up exercise again?

Sex hormones decline with age. In both men and women there is a slow and steady decline of testosterone, which leads to a drop in sexual libido and lean muscle mass. The drop in testosterone is also behind the slowing of metabolism that both women and men experience as they age. Testosterone plays a role in metabolism because it builds muscle, and muscles burn far more calories than fat does. You can, of course, play a role in building your muscles and preventing their atrophy by doing resistance exercises to strengthen your muscles. You lose the free ride of youth as you age and your testosterone declines, but that doesn't mean you have to sit back and let it happen.

Menopause

Menopause is defined as occurring one year after a woman's last period. The average age of menopause is 51, but the physiologic processes surrounding the ovaries' retirement usually begin when a woman is in her midforties. Perimenopausal symptoms start to occur in the five or so years before reaching menopause. These symptoms are a consequence of the ovaries becoming more erratic in their estrogen production. Symptoms consist of mood swings, memory difficulties, night sweats, hot flashes, vaginal dryness, irregular periods, and insomnia. There is a women can do to minimize these symptoms during this process.

Hot flashes can be minimized in some women by avoiding hot beverages, spicy food, alcohol, and caffeine and trying to minimize stressful situations. Some women find that adding soy to their diet diminishes hot flashes, but it's probably best to limit soy to only one or two servings a day, since some studies indicate that too much soy might promote some types of breast cancer. Hormones or nonhormonal medications are available if symptoms are debilitating, but most women can get by with simple lifestyle measures.

To combat insomnia and mood swings, get regular exercise, practice good stress management, get proper nutrition, and drink plenty of water. Prioritize which things really need to get done now and which are not essential. Have a bedtime ritual, and keep to a predictable schedule. Devote some time to relaxation and self-nurturing every day. For memory and brainpower, try to back down on multitasking, focus on one thing at a time, write things down, and exercise your brain daily with new, stimulating mental activities and challenges.

Also, remind yourself that things will get better. For many women, midlife is a great time of life, as they finally have time to focus on doing what they really like to do. Take it one day at a time, and try to keep your sense of humor. Talk to female friends about it, too, and share your experiences and ideas. You will always find other women who are eager to discuss their experiences with you.

As far as hormone replacement therapy is concerned, the current recommendation is as follows: if you are really miserable in the first few years after menopause, short-term, low-dose hormone therapy is an option. Hormone replacement should be considered a temporary replacement to ease your body through the transition. Some women, about 5 percent, do continue to have hot flashes in their later years. If this is the case for you, quality-of-life issues need to be weighed against the small but present increase in the risks of breast cancer, heart attacks, and blood clots with hormone replacement.

Benign Prostate Hyperplasia

Men also have a type of menopause as their testosterone wanes, but the process is much more subtle and gradual. Though men don't go through the turbulence of menopause as women do, they have their own issues. Men often gradually start to notice a slowing of the urinary stream as their prostate enlarges. Slow, gradual enlargement of the prostate gland is called benign prostate hyperplasia (BPH). Fifty percent of men have BPH by age 60, and 90 percent have it by age 85. Because the prostate gland wraps right around the urethra, its enlargement can interfere with urinating, so much that sleep becomes disrupted because it becomes necessary to urinate every two hours since the bladder never empties entirely. There are, of course, medications and procedures to fix this if it becomes a real nuisance; some men try herbs such as saw palmetto, though there isn't solid evidence that it helps significantly.

Osteoporosis

There is a one-in-two chance that a woman will have an osteoporosis-related fracture in her lifetime, and there is a one-in-four chance that a man will have an osteoporosis-related fracture in his lifetime. Hip fractures are the most serious. Twenty-five percent of those over 50 who experience a hip fracture die in the first year following the incident, and 20 percent lose their independence at home and have to move into an assisted living facility. Vertebral (spinal) fractures are twice as common as hip fractures and can be quite debilitating because they are so painful.

How can you keep your bones healthy and prevent osteoporosis? Prevention starts early in life. You reach your peak bone mass in your twenties, so during these years it is important to do a lot of weight-bearing exercise and get enough calcium and vitamin D. Building up strong bones in your teens and twenties pays off big-time later in life.

After age 30, for both men and women, bone mass undergoes a very slow, steady decline. Both estrogen and testosterone are important for maintaining bone mass. In women, bone mass takes a big drop in the years surrounding menopause, but then it levels off to a more gradual decline. Men have a slow decline throughout life; they don't have the big drop that women have at menopause, but they can get osteoporosis, too, particularly if they smoke, drink large amounts of alcohol, or have a low testosterone level.

Not getting enough calcium or vitamin D will contribute to the risk as well. You need calcium to build strong bones, and vitamin D is necessary to absorb calcium. Getting enough vitamin D and calcium becomes more of an issue in your later years because the body is less able to absorb calcium and manufacture the necessary vitamin D. Those who are at the highest risk for osteoporosis are thin, elderly Caucasian and Asian women who have a family history of osteoporosis. Various medical conditions or chronic use of certain medications can also increase the risk, as can smoking, alcohol, and inactivity.

What can you do to protect your bones? The best way to keep your bones strong is to do weight-bearing exercise, such as weight lifting, or any activity that works against gravity, such as running or even walking. Aim for at least 30 minutes each day. The exact amount of calcium and vitamin D needed is debated because, although both are necessary for strong bones, exercise is really the biggest player in bone health. Calcium is found in dairy foods and leafy dark green vegetables such as spinach. Vitamin D is mostly made from your skin after a brief exposure (20 minutes a day) to direct sunlight. The general recommendation for women, starting in their forties, is to take a calcium supplement, 1,200 milligrams per day, and a vitamin D supplement, 800 IU per day. If you have a high-risk profile, consider speaking to your doctor about getting screened for osteoporosis. Also, discuss hormone therapy (if you are a woman), or look into other bone-strengthening medications such as bisphosphonates.

The main message here is that exercise is by far the best way to maintain strong, healthy bones. Your bones will respond no matter what your age or whether you already have osteoporosis or not. It's never too late.

Protecting Your Hearing

One third of people over 65 have some degree of hearing loss. Some hearing loss is an unavoidable aspect of aging, but there is one major preventive measure you can do to minimize it: avoid loud noises.

The rate of hearing loss is on the rise, even in teenagers, especially those who use headphones when listening to loud music. *Loud noise kills the nerve cells of your inner ear, and they don't grow back.* These cells are crucial for translating sound waves into information your brain can understand. In aging, many of these cells will wear down, but loud noise accelerates the process significantly.

But how loud is loud? Sound is measured in decibels. A whisper is 30 decibels. Normal conversation is 60 decibels. A power lawn mower is 90 decibels. Rock concerts are 120 decibels. A shotgun blast or explosion is 140 decibels. Anything below 80 decibels (produced by a typical vacuum cleaner) is fine for the ears, but louder noises can cause the cells irreparable damage.

You can protect your ears from loud noises by wearing earplugs or earmuffs that typically can reduce noise by 15 to 30 decibels. Earplugs are better for lower frequencies and earmuffs for higher frequencies. Don't blast music on your headphones.

Don't smoke. In one study cigarette smokers were 70 percent more likely to lose their hearing than nonsmokers. Also, don't use cotton swabs to clean inside your ears. If you get wax buildup in your ears, use an earwax softener for a couple of days and then irrigate the wax out with a bulb syringe and lukewarm water.

Your hearing plays an important role in allowing you to engage in life fully. Protect it, and it will serve you well.

Protecting Your Vision

Every year, 50,000 Americans lose their vision. One third of these cases are preventable through proper lifestyle measures and early detection and treatment.

The three major causes of blindness are cataracts, macular degeneration, and glaucoma.

Cataracts occur due to a change in the chemical composition of the eye's lens, which causes the lens to become cloudy. This condition occurs in most people who live past 70, but frequent exposure to direct sunlight seems to accelerate the process. This condition can easily be treated with surgery to remove and replace the lens.

Macular degeneration is a condition in which the area of the retina involved in central vision, the macula, degenerates. Macular degeneration is the leading cause of blindness in people over age 55. Too much direct sunlight can accelerate the process. The retina is fed by small blood vessels, so conditions that cause arterial damage, such as high blood pressure, high cholesterol, smoking, and diabetes, all increase the risk of this condition. A diet high in fruits and vegetables that supplies a lot of anti-oxidants appears to decrease the risk of macular degeneration as well.

Glaucoma is a condition in which the optic nerve is damaged, often, but not always, due to high pressure within the eye. Pressure in the eye can occur if your eye makes too much fluid or fails to absorb it at the rate it is produced. Untreated glaucoma can lead to blindness. In general, routine eye checks are advised every two to four years between the ages of 40 and 64 and every year or two after 65.

You won't irreversibly harm your vision if you sit too close to the television, read with a dim light, or stare at a computer all day, although you will cause eye-strain. It is important, though, to wear UV light–protective sunglasses when in direct sun. You also need to protect the blood vessels that feed the retina of the eye by keeping your blood pressure, cholesterol, and blood sugar low and by not smoking. Your eyes are precious and serve a critical role in your ability to engage in an active, healthy lifestyle, so guard this treasure carefully.

Keeping Your Skin Healthy

As we age, we all start to see and feel changes in our skin. Some of these changes are natural, unavoidable, and harmless, but others, such as skin cancer, can be serious. All these changes can have a genetic component, but, more important, they have an environmental component, the most important one being the sun. Both skin cancer and premature aging are caused by sun exposure.

The most important thing you can do for your skin is to wear sunscreen every day. Sunscreens don't need to be expensive. They should be broad spectrum (blocking both UVA and UVB rays) and at least SPF 15. Sweatproof or waterproof products are helpful for sports or swimming, but like all sunscreens they need to be reapplied every few hours. Remember your sunglasses and lip protection as well!

Types of skin cancers include squamous cell, basal cell, and melanoma, which is the most serious skin cancer. If detected early, melanoma can be treated successfully. Excessive exposure to the sun and particularly sunburns are the most important preventable risk for melanoma. Other factors include genetics and immune deficiencies. You are at increased risk if you have red or blond hair, if you have many moles or atypical moles, and if you have a family history of melanoma.

A changing, new, or "different" mole requires immediate medical attention. The "ABCD rule" outlines the warning signs of melanoma:

A	*Asymmetry*	One half does not match the other half.
B	*Border irregularity*	The edges are ragged or blurred.
C	*Color*	The pigment is not uniform.
D	*Diameter*	Melanomas are usually (but not always) greater than 6 millimeter in diameter.

Everyone should examine his or her own skin on a regular basis and be aware of any lesions on the skin. Any new or changing growth should be brought to the attention of a physician. In addition, anyone with increased risk factors should get a regular skin examination. This includes those who have had a previous skin cancer or significant sun exposure/sunburn history and those with a high mole count, atypical moles, or a family history of melanoma.

If you can't remember anything else, remember this one key point: when it comes to taking care of your skin, the most important message is sunscreen, sunscreen, and sunscreen.

Preventive Care Guidelines

In addition to the cancer-screening guidelines we reviewed last week, the following preventive care services are recommended for adults:

- Blood work for cholesterol and fasting glucose should be done every three to five years (more frequently if you are in a higher risk category or if abnormalities have previously been discovered).

- Blood pressure should be checked at every medical visit.

- Bone density tests should be done in women as a baseline at menopause and then every three years if normal. If you fall in a higher risk category for osteoporosis or the prior bone density tests show osteopenia (thinning of the bone) or osteoporosis, every one to two years is recommended.

- Dental exams should be done one to two times per year to maintain healthy gums and teeth.

- Vision should be checked every three to five years under age 40 and every two to four years between ages 40 and 65. After age 65, yearly eye exams are recommended. If you have diabetes, you should get yearly eye exams regardless of your age. Glaucoma checks should be done yearly starting at age 65. If there is a family history of glaucoma or you are in a higher risk category such as African American, you should start getting yearly glaucoma checks at age 50.

- Check with your doctor at each yearly exam, to make sure you are up to date on adult vaccinations.

Vaccinations

A vaccination works by giving you a very small dose of a bacterium, virus, or toxin to prepare your immune system to quickly mobilize and fight in the event you are exposed to it in the future.

Staying up to date on vaccinations is an important way for you, as an adult, to stay healthy. A couple of decades ago, people became concerned that preservatives in vaccines might be the cause of a rise in the prevalence of autism. This concern has proven false, yet because these people did not get vaccinated or vaccinate their children, we are seeing a rise in some serious, previously rare diseases. Measles, for example, has been reported in growing numbers. If you don't have an up-to-date vaccination record, I urge you to create one now. You can keep your vaccination records online, for example, at Google Health or Microsoft Health Vault, in your own personal health record. Here are the vaccines recommended for adults. Assuming you had all your childhood vaccines:

- Make sure you have had two, not just one, **measles** vaccinations. The guidelines changed in the 1990s, when it became clear that people needed to have a second vaccine, but not everyone got the second shot. It is generally given as measles, mumps, rubella (MMR) combination vaccine.

- In addition to the **polio** shots you should have been given as a child, you should get one final booster sometime during adulthood; we usually give it before a patient travels abroad.

- Your **tetanus** vaccination should be updated every ten years. The tetanus vaccine usually has a couple of other vaccines in it, such as **diphtheria** and **pertussis** (whooping cough), so you get added protection from these diseases as well.

- You may have been vaccinated against **hepatitis B** in childhood, but check on this. This vaccine is given in a three-shot series.

- If you are traveling to a developing country, you will need **hepatitis A** vaccinations as well. This vaccine is given in a two-shot series. You can have hepatitis A and B combined into one vaccine to minimize the number of shots.

- If you are a woman under age 27, the human papillomavirus (**HPV**) vaccine is recommended to prevent cervical cancer. This is a three-shot series.

- If you have asthma, diabetes, or some other chronic disease that may lower your immunity, be sure to get one **pneumococcus** shot. If you get this shot before age 65, you'll be given a booster when you turn 65.

- Everyone should get the yearly flu vaccine unless he or she is allergic to eggs (with which they are prepared) or has some other contraindication.

- For travel abroad, you may also need **typhoid, yellow fever,** and **meningococcus** vaccinations. Children are often now routinely vaccinated against meningococcus.

- Finally, check to see whether you had the **varicella** (chicken pox) vaccine. If you had chicken pox as a child or if were born before 1957, you don't need this vaccine. (Those born before 1957 are presumed to have had chicken pox as a child.)

- **Herpes zoster** vaccine (which targets varicella recurrence, not herpes) is also now available to prevent shingles, a painful, localized rash caused by varicella. This is recommended to those over age 60.

Vaccinations are easy and go a long way toward keeping you healthy, so talk to your doctor if you aren't sure which ones you've received.

So there you go, a recipe on how to age. The recipe emphasizes all of the health messages you have been working on now for almost three months. Certainly, staying healthy is not always easy, but by now you see that behavior evolution—albeit slow—is really the path to improving much of your health. You can't force gene evolution, but you can practice a healthy lifestyle. Although you didn't have a say in which genes you were born with, you do have a say in whether those genes are turned on or off. And that's how you'll put yourself in the driver's seat of your health.

In the next section, I'll review how nutrition needs can change throughout life and whether or not it makes sense for you to take any vitamins, minerals, or other supplements. I'm not a big supplement fan. I think most supplements benefit only the sellers' pocketbooks, but there are a few that I think are not only helpful but can improve your health and extend your life span.

NUTRITION: VITAMINS AND MINERALS

In the past ten weeks, we've talked a lot about calories—calories from carbohydrates, calories from protein, calories from fat, and too many calories from simply overeating. Calories get the bulk of the attention because most people look at nutrition from the standpoint of wanting to lose weight, but food contains much more than just these three macronutrients and their calories. Food also contains vitamins, minerals, and other chemicals—some yet to be discovered—that are vital for health. These nutrients don't provide calories, but I'm going to show you what they do provide and why they are so important.

Vitamins are required in a variety of chemical reactions critical for sustaining life. Some vitamins are fat-soluble, including vitamins A, D, E, and K. These vitamins are not easily excreted, so they can reach toxic levels if you ingest too much. This usually happens only if you take large quantities of vitamin supplements.

The water-soluble vitamins are the B vitamins and vitamin C. These vitamins are easily excreted. I don't recommend megadoses of any vitamins or supplements, but if you do take megadoses of these vitamins, you will just urinate the excess amount out of your system.

Minerals are divided into major minerals and trace minerals. Minerals are used in nerve impulse transmission, muscle cell contractility, maintaining water balance, and building your body's physical structure. The major minerals are needed in much larger amounts than the trace minerals. If you are like most people, you probably haven't even heard of some of the trace minerals. They are needed in only very tiny amounts to get their job done.

MAJOR MINERALS

Calcium	Potassium
Chlorine	Sodium
Phosphorus	Sulfur

TRACE MINERALS

Arsenic	Manganese
Boron	Molybdenum
Cobalt	Nickel
Copper	Selenium
Chromium	Silicon
Fluorine	Vanadium
Iodine	Zinc
Iron	

Water makes up 60 percent of our body. So it is obviously a crucial element of our diet. How much water we need each day varies from person to person. You lose water each day in your urine, sweat, and bowel movements, and you also lose fluids from your respiratory tract when you breathe. The food you eat provides some of your water requirements, and liquids provide the rest. Any beverage you consume has water in it. Some beverage choices are obviously better than others. Plain old water is always a safe, healthful option. How much water should you drink each day? If your urine is dark yellow, you need to drink more fluids; if it is pale yellow, you are adequately hydrated.

Fruits and vegetables contain an additional class of nutrients called *phytochemicals*. Phytochemicals simply means "plant chemicals." Some phytochemicals, including certain vitamins, are antioxidants. As you already know, oxidizing agents (free radicals) are molecules hungry for electrons that snatch them away from any molecule they can find. These oxidizing bad boys snatch electrons from molecules in the cell membrane; they grab electrons from organelles within the cell; they even steal electrons from the cell's sacred DNA.

When a molecule loses electrons, it can become altered in a way that makes it dysfunctional. Good-guy antioxidants work by selflessly sacrificing their own electrons to the bad-guy oxidizing agents so that the vital cell structures won't be robbed of their electrons. Pretty clever, eh? Oxidizing agents come from the ultraviolet radiation of the sun, cigarette smoke, and pollution. Each one of your cells actually gets thousands of oxidative hits each day, so it is critical that you get an adequate supply of antioxidants. The health consequences of oxidation include cancer, heart disease, blindness from macular degeneration, and cataracts.

Where do we get antioxidants? We get them from fruits and vegetables. These are our major sources of antioxidants. Can we get them in a pill? Yes, we can get them in a pill, but unfortunately heart protection or cancer reduction has never been demonstrated when the antioxidant has been taken in pill form. There have been many attempts to test various antioxidants such as vitamins C and E, beta-carotene, and selenium to see whether they can counteract the consequences of oxidizing agents, but what has been found is that no *one* antioxidant can stand alone and do the job. In fact, if you look at where antioxidants work in a cell, they all maintain different positions, each fulfilling some sort of antioxidant-specific job description. Some antioxidants set up camp in the cell membrane, some perch themselves in the cytoplasm, and still others fearlessly guard the cell's precious DNA. They work as a team, and perhaps for this reason we have been unsuccessful in finding one single magic antioxidant bullet. For now there is no pill. You simply have to eat your fruits and vegetables, just as your mother said.

When might you need to supplement your diet with a vitamin or mineral? Most of the time, you get all that you need by simply eating a well-balanced diet. But there are a few circumstances in which you might want to consider taking a supplement.

- If you are a menstruating woman, particularly with a heavy flow, or if your diet is light in iron, you may want to supplement with an iron pill.

- If you don't eat many dairy products, you should supplement with calcium. Postmenopausal women should also supplement with calcium as well as vitamin D to protect against osteoporosis. The recommended dose is calcium, 1,200 milligrams per day, and vitamin D, 800 IU per day. Remember, though, that the most important proactive measure for osteoporosis is a regular exercise routine that involves weight-bearing activities.

- Recent studies demonstrate a link between low vitamin D levels and an increase in overall mortality. Vitamin D appears to offer a protective effect against cancer, although its exact mechanism of action is not known. Low vitamin D levels have also been associated with an increased risk of heart attacks. Vitamin D is toxic at high doses, but it appears that a large number of people have lower-than-normal vitamin D levels. It is thought that perhaps this is because more people are avoiding the sun, since vitamin D is made from a precursor in the skin that is activated by the sun.

- The most frequently recommended supplement today is omega-3 fatty acids, which improve triglyceride and HDL levels, decrease inflammation, and appear to decrease blood pressure. They also increase BDNF and so appear to be beneficial to memory and mood.

- If you are pregnant or trying to get pregnant, you should take prenatal vitamins including folic acid, which helps prevent neural tube birth defects.

- If you are breast-feeding, you may also want to take more iron, folic acid, and calcium.

- If you are a vegetarian, you may need extra vitamin B12, as this is found only in animal products. You may also need extra calcium, zinc, iron, and vitamin D (800 IU daily) if your eating preferences do not include any meat, dairy, or other animal products.

In any event, it is not a bad idea to take one standard multivitamin a day—just in case! So go ahead and swallow your multivitamin, and then start planning how to make sure you get the really important nutrients by eating your quota of fresh fruits and vegetables each day.

FITNESS: FITNESS AND AGING

Fitness is important to your health no matter how old you are. Your body's physiology does change as you age, but regardless of age, the same principles for fitness apply. You still need to do aerobic activity to keep your heart, lungs, and muscles strong and efficient. You still need to do resistance and flexibility exercises to keep your muscles strong and your tissues flexible.

One's cardiorespiratory capacity does decline a bit with age. Peak performance generally occurs in your twenties, with a slow steady decline throughout the rest of your life. But although some decline is inevitable, it can be small. For example, if you are a well-conditioned 80-year-old, you may not be able to surpass a 20- or 30-year-old who is in top athletic shape, but you are probably physiologically superior to many unconditioned 20- or 30-year-olds. Your personal VO$_2$ max (which is how much oxygen your body can utilize when you are working out at your maximum level) will be lower than what it was when you were younger, but if you stay in shape, it may remain better than most people's.

What about your muscles? They too decline after hitting a peak in your twenties. If you don't exercise your muscles regularly, they will start to atrophy on an ongoing basis throughout your life after you have hit your peak. This loss of muscle is what accounts for a slower metabolism as we age, and it is this reduction in metabolism that often results in a slow, gradual weight gain over the years. The good news, though, is that this does not need to happen, at least not to a large extent. Sure, you will have some reduction in muscle over your lifetime, but if you exercise your muscles regularly, you will keep them strong. If you use your muscles, you are telling your body that they are still important to you, so they should be preserved. The most important muscles to preserve in aging are your core muscles (i.e., your chest, abdomen, back, shoulders, and thigh muscles). For one thing, they are your largest muscles and will help you maintain a higher metabolism, but, more important, strong core muscles help people retain their balance and mobility. In the later years, this is one of the biggest determinants in deciding who is able to remain independent at home and who needs to be in an assisted living environment.

Balance also declines with age due to a reduction in nerve connections in the cerebellum as well as in the joints. These nerves are important because they give your brain valuable information about your position in space. The two best things a person can do to preserve balance are to keep the core muscles strong and to participate in tai chi or chi gong, which are slow, rhythmic Eastern movements that build strength and balance.

Finally, tendons and ligaments shorten and become less flexible with aging, so it is important to maintain flexibility with stretching exercises. Better flexibility means less stiffness, fewer injuries, and easier overall movement.

So here's the message: as you go through life and do that aging thing, remember, you're not off the hook as you get older. You still need exercise. In fact, you need it more than ever. No matter what your age, you will continue to get all of the same health benefits of exercise.

Arthritis

In the United States, arthritis is the most common form of disability. There are several different kinds of arthritic conditions, but the most commonly seen is degenerative arthritis, also known as osteoarthritis. Osteoarthritis represents half of all cases of arthritis and accounts for an estimated 70 million sick days in the workplace each year.

The causes of arthritis are partly wear and tear, or previous injury on a joint and partly genetics. Some people with a lot of wear and tear on a joint never get osteoarthritis, and some people who show significant osteoarthritis on X-ray never have symptoms. Women are more likely to have arthritis of the hands and knees, while men are more likely to have arthritis of the hips, knees, and spine.

In osteoarthritis, the cartilage that caps and protects the bones within a joint wears down. This exposes bone to bone, which is painful and also irritating to the soft tissues. Bone spurs (little stubs of new bone growth) form in response to this irritation, so that the joint gradually enlarges with bony growths. A low-grade inflammation develops in the surrounding soft tissues.

The best way to prevent arthritis is to avoid being overweight, since that puts stress on the joints of the lower body, particularly the knees. Also, try to avoid abnormal joint stress by wearing proper shoes and by keeping the muscles around the joints strong and well supported. Consider cross training to prevent any single exercise from constantly wearing on the same joints over and over.

If you already have arthritis, exercise will reduce the pain and disability, partly because it stimulates the production of synovial fluid that lubricates the joints. There's another good reason to stay active! When you have arthritis, you will have less pain if you move your joints frequently; if you are sedentary, your joints will become stiff and even more painful. You may need to switch to forms of exercise that are easier on the joints, such as swimming or bike riding. Regular daily exercise is also recommended in arthritis because it improves overall muscle tone and balance and thus helps remove strain on the joints.

Harry is 89 years old and an inspiration to all those who wish to age well. Harry did not have an easy life. He was raised in Iowa by an impoverished single mother. In his early twenties he was the pilot of a fighter plane that was shot down in World War II and was a prisoner of war for a year. After the war, he worked in a lumberyard for twenty years and was eventually able to buy the business with three other friends. Today, at the age of 89, Harry is as sharp and playful as any 30-year-old I have ever met. What is his secret? He has always been active, swimming, running, and, later in life, walking. He is involved in community groups and still enjoys reading for pleasure. He has a great sense of humor and a real love of life. Harry still travels around the world with his wife, Judy. They even take three-week-long road trips together. He is truly an inspiration and a model for healthy living.

Shirley lost her husband when she was 82. Her children brought her into The Program because they were worried about her living independently at home and wanted her to be as healthy as possible. Shirley began a fitness program where she worked on increasing her aerobic fitness as well as her balance, which had become a little shaky. Her family was very supportive; she continued to spend time with her daughters and grandchildren. She also got back into tutoring high school children. Eventually, she began to bloom again. She is now 85 and serves as another model for aging successfully.

LEARN IT!

- Your genes determine only 20 to 30 percent of how you age.

- Your brain can produce new neurons, even late in life, particularly if you exercise.

- Exercise improves your memory by causing your brain to produce BDNF, a chemical that promotes both new connections between nerve cells and the birth of new neurons.

- Exercise may improve your sex life because it enables your brain to produce more DHEA, the precursor of testosterone and estrogen, which declines with age.

- Antioxidants are in fruits and vegetables and protect your cells from the cancer-causing and aging effects of free radicals, so get plenty of fruits and vegetables in your diet.

- Stay at a lean weight because fat cells secrete chemicals that promote the aging process.

- Take a multivitamin every day and consult your doctor about whether you might benefit from other supplements.

PERSONALIZE IT!

This week, work on your Social Brain.

Your brain's physiology is designed for social, collaborative interactions. When you are around other people, your brain's chemicals change and your neural circuits fire in ways that let you learn from others' experiences. Take advantage of your social brain to learn from others and to get the collaboration and support you need to achieve your goals and stay healthy.

Here are some examples of how people in The Program have personalized this brain principle and put it into action.

- Laurie A., a 48-year-old mother of two, was a member of a book club that had met for ten years. These book club friends decided to do The Program together, and the book club served as the support network within which they all worked together to share their challenges and triumphs and brainstorm on ways they could work around their individual challenges.

- Sheri M., a 43-year-old single mother of two teenagers, incorporated her family into The Program and picked topics to discuss at dinner so the teenagers would learn the information, too. They all kept one another accountable for the goals they had set. Sheri says that if you want to be sure you will stick to your goals you should pick a teenager as your coach. Teenagers don't let you get away with anything!

- Renee T., a 25-year-old graphic artist, did The Program with her sister. They were already in the habit of talking to each other almost every day on the phone, so they became each other's personal coaches while they did The Program.

- Tom W., a 71-year-old retired investor, did The Program with his wife. They found it to be quite a bonding experience, since they began to talk more about issues of stress, mood, and what life really meant to them.

- Tim P., a 35-year-old salesman was not comfortable sharing his personal issues with others. He was having some problems at work and at home. He found a psychologist whom he used as his confidant and coach as he worked to improve his life and general health habits. This worked out really well for him.

LIVE IT!

- Review last week's goals and create this week's short-term goals.

- Identify the top things we discussed about successful aging that you believe you are doing really well. Now identify areas in which you feel you could improve.

- Look at the list of preventive care guidelines in this week's chapter and make sure you are up to date. If you aren't, make an appointment with your physician to discuss them. You can also check with your doctor to see whether your blood pressure, blood sugar, and cholesterol have improved now that you have had a new and better lifestyle for the past eleven weeks.

- Review the past eleven weeks of The Program and create a list of all the successes you have experienced so far. List all the strategies you have tried that worked. Note even the small victories, and keep track of the strategies that have been successful. Small changes can result in big outcomes over time.

- Review the past eleven weeks and think of times you fell down in one of your health goals but got right back up. One of the biggest predictors of your success in staying on track is your ability to get back on your feet quickly.

HEALTHY FOREVER

We are what we repeatedly do.
Excellence, then, is not an act, but a habit.

—ARISTOTLE

CONGRATULATIONS! This is the final week of The Program. By now, you know more about health and how your brain and body work than most people. As you prepare to move into the maintenance phase of a healthy lifestyle, I want to review a few important things with you.

First, keep in mind that as you go through the rest of your life following a healthy lifestyle, you'll probably find that you need to swim against the current of our culture. What is considered "normal" in today's world—"normal" food choices, "normal" portions, "normal" physical activity—is not really normal at all. These things are not normal according to what our genes have evolved to be able to handle. You need to get used to the idea that you will have to be somewhat *abnormal* if you want to stay healthy. I don't mean that you have to be militaristic about your new life and never have another dessert or miss a day of exercise. As I've said before, I'm all for following the 80/20 rule! But I do think you have to live somewhat defensively so that you aren't drawn right back into the lifestyle you had before you started The Program.

Also, never underestimate the role you can have in influencing those around you, particularly children. If you have kids, realize that the lifestyle they see you living is, for the most part, the kind of lifestyle they will adopt. Think about the habits you yourself grew up with. Although there are exceptions to this, for the most part, people tend to grow up emulating their parents' health habits. So whether in the realm of nutrition or exercise or simply the way you handle stress or balance in your life, understand that if you have kids, the health habits you show them by your example can affect them just as much as they affect you.

You can also make a difference in the health of the community around you. The skyrocketing number of people suffering from obesity, diabetes, and other lifestyle-related diseases underscores the need for all of us to take a more active role in our health. I am optimistic that the health care crisis we are currently in can be turned around in much the same way that the antismoking campaign of the 1970s convinced many millions of people to stop smoking. But it depends on us—getting the word out, educating ourselves and others, and providing support for change.

> Be the change you want to see in the world.
> —MAHATMA GANDHI

Sometime during the past twelve weeks, you may have become bored with your "health project." Perhaps you got tired of keeping track of what you ate and how much exercise you managed to do. Guess what? This is part of the process, too. Living a healthy lifestyle is not always exciting, fun, or interesting. It just "is." You need to get past the fact that some of it can be boring, because anything you do over and over can become tedious. But this does not mean you should not do it.

I hope you have found some joy in moving your body daily. I hope you miss your exercise routine when you don't manage to get it in. But if that's not the case, I hope you will keep on doing it anyway.

Do you need to be perfect? Of course not, but you do need to understand that everything that has to do with your health is interconnected: what you eat, how much you move, how well you sleep and handle stress, even your mood. It all matters. And, most important, *You have the biggest say in all these aspects of your health.* That's the main message of The Program: you play the leading role in the story of your health.

Healthful Family Eating

The ever-increasing numbers of children with obesity and type 2 diabetes have led health care professionals to predict that the children of today are likely to have a shorter life span than their parents. Imagine that! Health care professionals are urging parents to help reverse this trend by making family mealtimes a priority, a time when kids can learn about proper portion sizes and parents can encourage healthful behavior through their own example.

The family table offers many health benefits. According to recent research, kids who eat family dinners frequently not only tend to eat more healthfully, they are more likely to do well in school and less apt to get involved with drugs. The family table also promotes family bonding. This is a time to talk, listen, and create family memories. Here are some helpful hints about how you can eat healthfully as a family.

- Try to have one meal as a family at least once a day. It can even be breakfast!

- If your family is always "on the go," designate family dinner nights.

- Find recipes that are easy to make. Spend your time with the family, not in the kitchen.

- Turn off the television, and avoid answering the phone during the meal. Make family mealtime the top priority.

- Eat around a table, not side by side at a counter. Eating around a table is better for conversation and eye contact.

- Keep family mealtime positive, a time that everyone enjoys. Save disciplinary or uncomfortable conversations for another time when possible.

Eating together as a family is the best way to teach children healthy eating habits for a lifetime, but as I've indicated above, the benefits of eating together as a family extend far beyond this.

NUTRITION: WEIGHT LOSS MAINTENANCE

Most experts agree that keeping weight off after you have lost it is harder than losing the weight in the first place. There are several reasons for this. One, people tend to experience diet fatigue after they have been on a diet. They are able to maintain their enthusiasm for a diet in the short run, but after a while, they get tired of paying such close attention to what they are eating and not being able to enjoy whatever they want. What's more, *people who have lost weight need fewer calories to sustain that lower weight.* Generally, for each pound you lose, you need eight fewer calories per day to maintain your new weight. Often, the increased exercise and muscle mass from a good exercise program have increased your resting metabolism to compensate for some of the energy gap. But chances are that if you've lost a significant amount of weight, you are going to need to stay at a lower calorie level just to maintain your new, lower weight.

At first, the statistics in the field of weight loss maintenance can sound discouraging. Most studies show that of those who lose more than 10 percent of their body weight, only 20 percent keep it off for one year and only 5 percent keep it off for three years. The truth is, though, that these statistics reflect research studies whose participants are often much more difficult to treat than the average person. Many people who sign up for a research program do so because nothing else has worked. Studies that retrospectively ask people randomly whether they have lost and maintained 10 percent or more of their body weight show much higher success rates, as high as 65 percent! So the odds of successful maintenance are probably somewhere in between.

The National Weight Control Registry (www.nwcr.ws) was founded in 1994 to enroll and study people who have been successful in keeping weight off once they've lost it. The participants currently include more than four thousand people who have maintained at least a 30-pound weight loss for a year or longer. One study of a sample of this population looked at people who had lost more than 60 pounds and maintained it for more than five years. Here are the behavioral strategies these successful weight losers followed:

- They exercised on a regular basis, averaging about an hour a day.

- They watched the amount of fat in their diet.

- They weighed themselves at least once a week.

- They frequently continued to log their food intake.

- They ate breakfast in the morning.

- They maintained consistent eating patterns on both weekdays and weekends.

A different study looking at other successful weight loss maintainers showed that they had these characteristics in common:

- A high internal locus of control (that is, they were motivated by internal, not external, factors)

- High self-efficacy (that is, they *believed* they could do it)

- Better coping strategies for dealing with stress

- Good social support

This study also suggested that when weight loss had been maintained for more than two years, maintenance became quite a bit easier.

Yet another study focused on characteristics commonly found in weight regainers:

- They had not been satisfied with the amount of weight they had lost to begin with.

- They tended to evaluate their self-worth in terms of their shape and weight.

- They typically had a dichotomous, "on a diet, off a diet" way of thinking.

- They often used food to regulate their mood.

This is what I recommend to help you keep weight off once you have lost it:

- **Weigh yourself every morning.** Give yourself a three-pound window within which to fluctuate. Within that range, don't panic. Fluid shifts can easily account for fluctuations of three pounds. But do weigh yourself every morning or at least a few times a week. Weight tends to creep up slowly over time, so if you aren't keeping a close eye on it on a regular basis, it can happen without your noticing.

- **If you exceed the three-pound limit, start keeping a log of your daily food and exercise again.** Review all the tools you have learned in this program and focus on being more diligent until you get back to your target weight. If you jump back into a more vigilant mode as soon as you cross the three-pound limit, you should get back to your target weight in no time.

- **Take care of emotional issues,** since these do tend to influence weight control. Effective management of stress, anxiety, and depression will not only help your overall health, it will optimize your weight loss maintenance efforts as well.

- **Finally, and most important, exercise regularly.** I know, I know, I've said it so often before, but it is really true. Consistent physical activity is probably *the* most important factor in long-term weight loss maintenance. Among national weight control registrants, walking is the most popular activity, followed by cycling, weight lifting, and aerobics. The amount of time typically spent exercising by those who are maintaining weight loss is about 40 minutes a day.

The bottom line to all of this is that weight maintenance requires diligence on your part. You can ease up a little here and there, but the same principles of healthful eating and healthful living still apply. You can't lose weight and then go right back to your old ways of operating. You'll simply gain it all back. You have all the tools now not to only keep the weight you've lost off but to live the rest of your life in a healthy, vital way.

Remember that new lifestyle habits don't become permanent overnight or even after twelve weeks. You need to continue to work on them, constantly repeating your new behavior so that your brain eventually accepts this behavior as the way things should be. This is key. I've heard statements such as "It takes three weeks to make a habit." If it were that easy to make permanent lifestyle changes, think how healthy our world would be! For something as major as what you are trying to do, it takes far longer than a few weeks to make the changes permanent. It actually takes more like a year or two. And even after that, you are going to need to pay attention for the rest of your life because, unless our culture changes dramatically, you'll find large food portions, tempting, unhealthful food choices, and sedentary jobs will continue to be a part of our life landscape.

Also, I encourage you to try to keep plugged into a healthy social network, whether with family, friends, or work colleagues. If you haven't done so already, go to www.theprogrambook.com to find a variety of ways you can maintain your successes and keep living healthy. Think carefully about your personalized plans for maintenance. Continue to work on being your own best coach. The more support you create for yourself, the more likely you are to be successful in continuing your new, healthful habits for the rest of your life.

FITNESS: IT'S A MARATHON, NOT A SPRINT

This final section focuses on how to maintain a regular exercise program. This is an appropriate topic for The Program to end on because physical activity is probably the biggest determining factor in your health. As I keep saying, physical activity influences every aspect of your health, whether it is weight control, stress, sleep, mood, or risks for diabetes, cancer, and heart disease. Exercise also plays a huge role in how well you age. In fact, many experts say that if there is a fountain of youth, it is exercise.

By now I'm sure most of you have established a solid workout regimen, and you've probably come to miss it when you don't exercise for a few days. But even the most avid exercisers get pulled off their regimen now and then. Don't beat yourself up for slipping off the wagon. It's going to happen. The trick, as I've said many times, is to get right back into it.

Here are twenty tips for keeping physical activity in your routine despite your busy, hectic schedule.

1 **Choose activities you like.** Have fun when you exercise. Don't create a workout that is so onerous that you dread doing it.

2 **Vary your activities over the years so you don't get bored.** Don't feel that you have to stick to one and only one routine.

3 **Exercise with a buddy so you have someone who depends on you to show up,** someone who will keep you accountable and can add some social pleasure while you work out.

4 **Join an exercise class.** This provides some structure as well as expertise. You'll also benefit from the energy of those working out around you.

5 **If you like to exercise alone, keep it fun** by listening to music or books on tape, or simply use it as downtime to reflect and think without interruptions.

6 **Incorporate exercise into your social routine.** Meet a friend for a walk instead of for lunch.

7 If you find it hard to carve out time for exercise because of a busy work schedule, **do walk-and-talk meetings.** You can start a new trend in your corporate culture. Have coworkers keep a pair of walking shoes at the office, and take a walk when you need to meet. This way, you can take care of work issues, get a breath of fresh air, and get your exercise in at the same time.

8 Is there a time of day you need to check in with a loved one or catch up on some phone calls that don't require you to be sitting at your desk? **Take your cell phone for a walk**—get a headset and catch up on calls while you exercise.

9 **Set a future goal** by enrolling in a 10k race or a similar event. Planned, future events like this can be good motivators to keep you on track.

10 **Have a friendly competition with your spouse, friends, or work colleagues.** Challenge one another to exercise at least five days a week for half an hour. Mark it on a central calendar and have a reward at the end for all who are able to accomplish this goal.

11 If you have young kids who can't be left home alone while you exercise, **consider getting a treadmill.** You don't have to spend a lot of money for it; there is a lot of used exercise equipment for sale. Then you can watch your favorite TV show while you work out, or you can record your favorite shows so that you can replay them at a workout time that is more convenient for you. You can also get a small portable DVD player and watch movies or reruns of old TV shows on DVD.

12 If your day always seems to get away from you and you can't fit in time to exercise, try **doing it in the morning.** Lay out your workout clothes and shoes beside your bed so that you can get up, throw on your clothes, and go. Exercising in the morning is a good idea for those of you with busy lives in which free moments often disappear.

13 If you can't imagine fitting exercise into your morning, **schedule exercise into your day.** At work, put exercise into your schedule just as you would a meeting. If you work at home, schedule it in your day planner and honor it just as you would any other commitment. You can go for a walk. And remember, three ten-minute sessions of activity are fine for the thirty minutes of activity (the minimum you should do each day). You can also get a treadmill or stationary bike for your office and do three ten-minute sessions a day as a break between tasks to both clear your mind and get in your exercise.

14 If you have young children at home who can't be left alone, **hire a teenager to watch them for an hour** or have your spouse keep an eye on them while you do your workout.

15 You can also **join a gym that offers child care,** or you can take your kids along for a walk or run with a jogging stroller.

16 If your kids are old enough to ride their bikes along with you when you run, let them come with you. **Incorporate your family into your workout sessions** so you get in family time as well as exercise time. Bike, hike, or swim together.

17 For some people, **having a personal trainer is the answer.** This offers structure, accountability, and trained expertise to help you achieve a higher level of fitness.

18 **Join a gym.** Take advantage of the classes offered, the various equipment, and the personal trainers.

19 If you like physical activity for the camaraderie or competition found in sports, **join a local team or league.**

20 **Post a monthly exercise calendar in a prominent place** that you see daily to remind yourself of how frequently you are exercising. This is a helpful way to stay honest with yourself and really see how much exercise you get over the long run.

These are just a few tricks that have worked well for people in The Program. I'm sure you can add to this list. Decide which strategies resonate with you.

Since you are at the end of The Program, it's time to fill out your Health Risk Assessment Questionnaire (page 42) and Health Stats (page 370) again, and review your long- and short-term goals. How did you do? Did you make any progress? If you completely fulfilled your long-term goals, *great,* but remember that any motion in the right direction is reason to celebrate. Small changes *will* result in big outcomes over time.

Review all of the coaching principles we discussed in Week 2. For the statements on the next page give yourself a score from 1 to 5 on how well you feel you have been able to incorporate these coaching tips into your efforts toward living a healthy life: 1 = strongly disagree, 2 = disagree, 3 = mixed feelings, 4 = agree, 5 = strongly agree.

ARE YOU YOUR OWN BEST COACH?

1 I am entirely capable of changing for the better.

2 I am resilient. I know I can get through hard times and emerge even stronger.

3 I can usually see a silver lining in even the worst situation.

4 I am solely responsible for my behavior.

5 I am good at developing strategies to handle difficult situations or challenges.

6 I can identify the stage I am in right now when it comes to living healthfully.

7 I know how to take general information and personalize it so it works in my own individual life.

8 I know how to visualize my goals.

9 I know that living a healthy lifestyle does not require me to be perfect.

10 I am comfortable with gradual change as the way to achieve healthy sustainable behaviors.

Your total score on this quiz is not as important as how you scored on the individual statements. Did you improve in any of the coaching principles? Usually people feel they have in at least one or two areas. Which coaching principles come naturally to you? Which ones are more difficult? Are there any categories to which you responded with a 3 or less? Any statement in which you scored a 3 or less will indicate areas you will need to pay special attention to in the maintenance phase of The Program.

Decide what you would like to do now that the first twelve weeks of The Program are coming to an end. After all, the pursuit of a healthy, happy life never really ends. Think about whether you want to create a few new long-term goals for the *next* twelve weeks. Maintaining what you have achieved is certainly a goal in itself. And the techniques you've learned here about goal setting and being your own best coach can be applied to anything in your life—career, relationships, anything, it doesn't have to be specific to your health.

As you move forward, don't forget the importance of how your brain intrinsically operates. Now you know how to capitalize on the natural workings of your brain so that it will work for you and not against you.

LEARN IT!

- To stay healthy, you usually need to swim against the current of our society.

- Your behavior, like it or not, does influence those in your home and community.

- You are absolutely capable of maintaining weight loss but it does take effort. Weigh yourself daily or weekly, exercise regularly, watch your portions, and if you stray above 3 pounds over your maintenance weight, go back to keeping a food and exercise log. Pay attention to stress, sleep, and mood.

- Even the most avid of athletes falls off the exercise bandwagon now and then. Have a list of tricks to get yourself quickly back on track. Exercise delivers the biggest benefit of all to your health.

PERSONALIZE IT!

This week, celebrate your Adaptable Brain.

Your brain is capable of substantial change. At any age, you can learn, you can grow, and you can improve your skills for living a happier, healthier life.

Here are some examples of how people in The Program have personalized this brain principle and put it into action.

- Kyle M., a 46-year-old grocery manager, had to stop going to the movies because at 349 pounds he could no longer fit into the seats. He also had sleep apnea, drank too much alcohol, and felt depressed much of the time. On his thirty-ninth birthday he decided that he had had enough. He gave up alcohol, started walking the few miles to work every day, and began to pay attention to his food choices and portions. It wasn't easy because he struggled with binge eating and also experienced some setbacks with depression, but he worked with a counselor and slowly made progress. Three years later, by his forty-second birthday, he had lost 135 pounds. Kyle has maintained this weight loss for four years. When I asked Kyle what secret lay behind his amazing drive to accomplish his goals, he said simply, "I just decided I wanted to change." And so he did.

- Sheri B., now 31 years old, had struggled with drugs since age 13. At the bright young age of 21 she felt her life was ruined. She didn't know how to work in a regular job (she sold drugs to make her living), and she certainly didn't know how to live a healthy life. But Sheri didn't want her life to be this way, and she, too, decided to change. She saw her doctor, who helped her get into a rehabilitation program. She moved to a different county and got a job as a waitress in a restaurant. Although she was extremely shy, she developed friendships with her new colleagues, who played a critical role as her social support. She also started exercising every day to lift her spirits (and you know by now that this helped increase the dopamine levels in her brain, making it easier to stay off the drugs). Making these changes required Sheri to change her behavior in almost every part of her life. But, hard as that was, she did change. And she has now been drug-free for ten years.

- Jimmy E., a 33-year-old data programmer, felt stressed all the time and hated his job. His unhappiness and irritability began to affect his relationships both at home and at work. Jimmy decided to see a counselor and began to work on some of the Happiness Strategies detailed in Week 8. Over many, many months, he became a much happier man who was clearly more at peace with himself and his life. In fact, he became really quite witty and fun to be around. Through conscious effort, Jimmy had learned how to apply new, positive ways of thinking and coping, and over time this new way of thinking started to come quite naturally to him. It came naturally because, as you know, with time his brain physically changed and adjusted to his new way of living and thinking.

LIVE IT!

- Keep up your support network.

- Make goals even if just to maintain your progress.

- Remember, you don't need to be perfect. Follow the 80/20 rule.

- Remember to address all aspects of your health—that is, nutrition, activity, stress, sleep, and mood—because they are all interconnected.

- Your brain holds the key to a lot of your behavior, and you can use this to your advantage.

I hope you have enjoyed The Program and found it useful. Everyone deserves a happy, healthy life, and you should now have all the tools you need to bring good health and happiness into your own life. Remember, you are largely in the driver's seat when it comes to your health. There is so much you can do to stay healthy and happy. Your brain knows this, and so do I.

APPENDIX

- Putting It All Together

- Food Log

- Goals Log

- BMI Chart

- Health Stats

- Interpreting Your Health Stats

PUTTING IT ALL TOGETHER: HOW TO USE YOUR BRAIN FOR THE HEALTHIEST YOU

Your Selective Brain

Your brain does not consciously process all of the information it is exposed to on a daily basis; it is selective. Selective attention allows your brain to think while being on autopilot, thereby letting you do something else; but it can also allow unhealthy behaviors without your being aware of them. Change often starts by simply paying close attention to whatever behavior you would like to change.

CONCRETE WAYS TO APPLY THIS BRAIN PRINCIPLE

1 Track whatever behavior you are trying to modify so that you consciously pay more attention to this behavior.

2 Build in set reminders during the day to remind yourself to track your behavior so you get in the habit of doing it. You can set a watch alarm, set up a daily automatic text message, or send an e-mail reminder. Perhaps you and a friend can call each other every day to check in.

3 Keep your goals constantly in front of you. For example, have your goals appear as your computer's screen saver or keep them on a notepad in your car so that you see them every time you drive.

Your Resistant Brain

Although your brain can change, it is generally set up to resist change, especially sudden change. People who are ultimately successful in initiating and maintaining major behavioral changes usually make the changes one step at a time.

CONCRETE WAYS TO APPLY THIS BRAIN PRINCIPLE

1 Change slowly, advancing in a gradual stepwise progression. This is generally less stressful on the brain.

2 Try changing within some form of structure so you do not have to make decisions every step of the way. This requires less work for your brain.

3 People often fear unfamiliar or unknown situations, so try to have as much clarity and transparency as possible in whatever you are working toward. When people know the rules and know what is expected of them, they generally feel less stressful.

Your Emotional Brain

The rational and emotional centers of your brain are tightly interconnected. This means your emotions can influence your behavior, and that can be either good or bad. You can learn how to modify your mood and stress levels in positive ways through various well-defined behaviors that improve your ability to stay healthy and happy.

CONCRETE WAYS TO APPLY THIS BRAIN PRINCIPLE

1 Learn how to turn off negative emotions. For example, take some slow, deep breaths. Do regular exercise. Focus mentally on all of the positive things in your life for which you are grateful.

2 Do simple things that activate your pleasure centers. Listen to music. Read a book. Watch a comedy. Talk to a friend. Get a massage. Take a relaxing, hot bath.

3 Don't necessarily avoid stress. It's okay to challenge yourself outside of your comfort zone; challenges can help you grow stronger and better. It is more important to learn how to be able to turn the stress response off at will than to avoid stress altogether.

Your Rational Brain

The human brain, specifically your frontal cortex, is highly developed for problem-solving. You can use this problem-solving talent to strategize around the various challenges that come up when you are trying to practice healthy habits. You can also use your frontal cortex to better understand why you behave the way you do, and then you can consciously work to substitute healthy behaviors for unhealthy ones. Finally, you can use your Rational Brain to connect back to your Emotional Brain to modulate your mood or stress level.

CONCRETE WAYS TO APPLY THIS BRAIN PRINCIPLE

1 Identify challenges you anticipate will arise as you work toward your goals. For each challenge, devise a strategy to let you work around it. Because your Rational Brain is so tightly connected to your Emotional Brain, accomplishing your goals is more about problem-solving than about brute-force willpower.

2 Spend time understanding why you behave the way you do in certain situations. For example, if you feel you are reacting emotionally in ways you wish to change, practice replacing old thoughts and behaviors with new ones. Over time, your frontal cortex will develop new alternate paths of thought that become reflexive.

3 Remember to repeat new behaviors and thoughts over and over. Repetition is necessary for creating new physical circuits in the brain.

Your Believing Brain

Your brain is greatly influenced by whether or not you believe you can do something. In fact, simply believing in your ability to perform a task is as important as having the actual skill for doing it. Your brain promotes a lot of behavior that simply reflects who you think you are. Use this to your advantage. Break large goals into small steps that you can achieve, and this will gradually build your confidence. Also, always believe in your best self because, chances are, this is who you will become.

CONCRETE WAYS TO APPLY THIS BRAIN PRINCIPLE

1 You can learn to believe in yourself more by achieving success in small, little goals that lead up to your larger goal.

2   You will be more likely to believe in yourself if you surround yourself with people who have succeeded in a same or similar goal.

3   Stay positive. The thoughts you tell yourself often become a self-fulfilling prophecy, so if you find yourself thinking negative messages about yourself, stop and focus on what you are doing well.

4   Mentally rehearse (goal visualize) achieving your goal over and over to get your mind used to being at this end point.

Your Unique Brain

No two brains are the same. Everyone is born with unique blueprints of DNA, and everyone enjoys different life experiences. So, although the basic principles for staying healthy are the same for everyone, you need to choose how to make these principles work for you in your own personal life.

CONCRETE WAYS TO APPLY THIS BRAIN PRINCIPLE

1   Personalize healthy lifestyle behaviors so that they work for you in your own individual life. No one is the same, and there is no one-size-fits-all for how you apply these general brain principles to your life.

2   Understand that your needs in life may change over time so that behaviors may need to be modified. Stay flexible.

3   Listen to others about what strategies have worked for them so you can get new ideas and tips, but remember to modify their strategies to fit your needs.

Your Learning Brain

Your brain has a tremendous capacity to learn. Enhance factors that optimize learning. That is, get adequate sleep, minimize stress, and exercise regularly. Remember to repeat over and over whatever you want your brain to memorize. Your brain is also playful. It loves puzzles, humor, and questions. Finally, don't be afraid to make mistakes. Your brain learns from them, so they are an important part of growing.

CONCRETE WAYS TO APPLY THIS BRAIN PRINCIPLE

1 Your brain learns best when conditions are optimal for learning. You must get adequate sleep to learn optimally, and you must learn how to manage stress well. Stress reduces the blood flow and activity within the frontal cortex, the area of the brain that controls higher learning and problem-solving.

2 Exercise! Physically challenging your body releases all sorts of wonderful chemicals that ultimately grow your brain and increase your ability to learn and think creatively.

3 Mistakes are opportunities to learn. Your brain modifies itself when you make a mistake, so mistakes are not necessarily bad. They can allow growth.

Your Exercising Brain

Exercise changes both the function and physical structure of the brain. It increases numerous chemicals in both the brain and the body—chemicals that elevate mood, decrease stress, and increase mental alertness. Physical exercise also significantly increases brain activity, facilitating learning and memory. Exercise is your biggest ally in health *and* in behavior change because it optimizes the performance of both the body and the brain.

CONCRETE WAYS TO APPLY THIS BRAIN PRINCIPLE

1 Try to do thirty minutes of heart-pounding activity each day to keep your brain alert, creative, and learning optimally.

2 Incorporate more body movement into your day, in general. For example, walk to your errands at lunch. Take the stairs instead of the elevator.

3 If mood, sleep, and stress are issues you would like to improve, exercise is your biggest ally. It will change your brain physiologically to improve all three of these areas.

Your Motivated Brain

Your behavior is influenced by a chemical called dopamine. This chemical is released by "pleasure centers" in your brain, and it captures your attention and drives your motivation toward a behavior. Learn to structure your healthy behaviors around simple, healthy things that you enjoy. In this way, you can promote motivation and structure a lifestyle that is not only healthy but sustainable.

CONCRETE WAYS TO APPLY THIS BRAIN PRINCIPLE

1 Define the simple activities in life that can bring you joy (such as hiking in a park, listening to music, getting a massage), and make sure you incorporate these simple pleasures into your healthy lifestyle routines so that you are more likely to do them.

2 Have simple, healthy ways to reenforce healthy lifestyle behaviors. For example, after you do your exercise, you can reward yourself by allowing yourself to relax and read.

3   Avoid unhealthy behaviors (like drugs, alcohol, tobacco, and overeating) that might temporarily bring you joy but will ultimately impair your health.

Your Responsive Brain

Your health is not predestined by your genes, because the environment can turn genes on and off. Your brain responds profoundly to its surrounding environment. When you learn how to optimize your environment, you learn how to turn genes on or off, and for many genes, this can translate into behavior. It is critical to set up your world so that it encourages healthy living.

CONCRETE WAYS TO APPLY THIS BRAIN PRINCIPLE

1   Your brain responds chemically to its surrounding environment, affecting which genes are turned on and off. Optimize your physical world so that it promotes the behavior you want. Keep healthy food in and junk food out of the house. Keep workout clothes in plain view so that you are encouraged to exercise.

2   Your brain responds to your social environment. Surround yourself with friends who model behavior you like; minimize interactions with those who have behaviors you are trying to avoid.

3   In order to stay healthy in today's world, you will always need to be vigilant, because many in our current society are not living with particularly healthy habits. In order to live healthfully, you will probably need to live a little differently from those around you.

Your Social Brain

Your brain's physiology is designed for social, collaborative interactions. When you are around other people, your brain's chemicals change and your neural circuits fire in ways that let you learn from other people's experiences. Take advantage of your Social Brain to learn from others and to get the collaboration and support you need to achieve your goals and stay healthy.

CONCRETE WAYS TO APPLY THIS BRAIN PRINCIPLE

1   Listen to others who share similar goals and learn from their experiences; share your stories with them as well. We can all learn from each other.

2   Cooperate and collaborate with others to reach your goals. We are intrinsically wired as humans to be social and collaborative.

3   Surround yourself with a positive, affirming social circle, as this can play a key role in keeping you strong and resilient when times get tough.

Your Adaptable Brain

Your brain is capable of substantial change. At any age, you can learn, you can grow, and you can improve your skills for living a happier, healthier life.

CONCRETE WAYS TO APPLY THIS BRAIN PRINCIPLE

1   It's good to push your brain out of its comfort zone—to learn, to grow stronger, and to adapt.

2   You can choose an area of the brain and intentionally grow that one specific area.

3   There is no time in your life that you stop growing and adapting. The best way to grow is to continually stimulate yourself physically and mentally.

FOOD LOG

Date _____

FOOD NAME   FOOD GROUP AND AMOUNT

Morning Time	Grains/ Starches	Veggies	Fruits	Dairy	Meats/ Substitute	Fats	Sweets

COMMENTS

Noon Time	Grains/ Starches	Veggies	Fruits	Dairy	Meats/ Substitute	Fats	Sweets

COMMENTS

Evening Time	Grains/ Starches	Veggies	Fruits	Dairy	Meats/ Substitute	Fats	Sweets

COMMENTS

Total number of servings in each category	Grains/ Starches	Veggies	Fruits	Dairy	Meats/ Substitute	Fats	Sweets

GOALS LOG

LONG-TERM GOALS

1 _____

2 _____

3 _____

SHORT-TERM GOALS

	Goals	Successes	Challenges and Strategies to Try

WEEK ONE

	Goals	Successes	Challenges and Strategies to Try
1			
2			
3			

WEEK TWO

	Goals	Successes	Challenges and Strategies to Try
1			
2			
3			

WEEK THREE

	Goals	Successes	Challenges and Strategies to Try
1			
2			
3			

WEEK FOUR

	Goals	Successes	Challenges and Strategies to Try
1			
2			
3			

WEEK FIVE

	Goals	Successes	Challenges and Strategies to Try
1			
2			
3			

	Goals	Successes	Challenges and Strategies to Try

WEEK SIX

1			
2			
3			

WEEK SEVEN

1			
2			
3			

WEEK EIGHT

1			
2			
3			

WEEK NINE

1			
2			
3			

WEEK TEN

1			
2			
3			

WEEK ELEVEN

1			
2			
3			

WEEK TWELVE

1			
2			
3			

BMI CHART

	Normal						Overweight				Obese						
BMI	**19**	**20**	**21**	**22**	**23**	**24**	**25**	**26**	**27**	**28**	**29**	**30**	**31**	**32**	**33**	**34**	**35**
HEIGHT (FEET/INCHES)	BODY WEIGHT (POUNDS)																
4'10"	91	95	100	105	110	115	119	124	129	134	138	143	148	153	158	162	167
4'11"	94	99	104	109	114	119	124	128	133	138	143	148	153	158	163	168	173
5'0"	97	102	107	112	118	123	128	133	138	143	148	153	158	164	169	174	179
5'1"	100	106	111	116	121	127	132	137	143	148	153	158	164	169	174	180	185
5'2"	104	109	115	120	125	131	136	142	147	153	158	164	169	175	180	186	191
5'3"	107	113	118	124	130	135	141	146	152	158	163	169	175	180	186	192	197
5'4"	110	116	122	128	134	140	145	151	157	163	169	174	180	186	192	198	203
5'5"	114	120	126	132	138	144	150	156	162	168	174	180	186	192	198	204	210
5'6"	117	124	130	136	142	148	155	161	167	173	179	185	192	198	204	210	216
5'7"	121	127	134	140	147	153	159	166	172	178	185	191	198	204	210	217	223
5'8"	125	131	138	144	151	158	164	171	177	184	190	197	203	210	217	223	230
5'9"	128	135	142	149	155	162	169	176	182	189	196	203	209	216	223	230	237
5'10"	132	139	146	153	160	167	174	181	188	195	202	209	216	223	230	236	243
5'11"	136	143	150	157	165	172	179	186	193	200	207	215	222	229	236	243	250
6'0"	140	147	155	162	169	177	184	191	199	206	213	221	228	235	243	250	258
6'1"	144	151	159	166	174	182	189	197	204	212	219	227	234	242	250	257	265
6'2"	148	155	163	171	179	187	194	202	210	218	225	233	241	249	256	264	272
6'3"	152	160	168	176	184	192	200	208	216	224	232	240	247	255	263	271	279
6'4"	156	164	172	180	189	197	205	213	221	230	238	246	254	262	271	279	287

Source: Adapted from *Clinical Guidelines on the Identification, Evaluation, and Treatment of Overweight and Obesity in Adults: The Evidence Report.*

*Surgery Indicated: BMI >35 with comorbidity; BMI >40 (Per 1991 NIH Conference Criteria)

Extreme Obesity

36	37	38	39	40	41	42	43	44	45	46	47	48	49	50	51	52	53	54
172	177	181	186	191	196	201	205	210	215	220	224	229	234	239	244	248	253	258
178	183	188	193	198	203	208	212	217	222	227	232	237	242	247	252	257	262	267
184	189	194	199	204	209	215	220	225	230	235	240	245	250	255	261	266	271	276
190	195	201	206	211	217	222	227	232	238	243	248	254	259	264	269	275	280	285
196	202	207	213	218	224	229	235	240	246	251	256	262	267	273	278	284	289	295
203	208	214	220	225	231	237	242	248	254	259	265	270	276	282	287	293	299	304
209	215	221	227	233	238	244	250	256	262	267	273	279	285	291	296	302	308	314
216	222	228	234	240	246	252	258	264	270	276	282	288	294	300	306	312	318	324
223	229	235	241	247	253	260	266	272	278	284	291	297	303	309	315	322	328	334
229	236	242	248	255	261	268	274	280	287	293	299	306	312	319	325	331	338	344
236	243	249	256	263	269	276	282	289	295	302	308	315	322	328	335	341	348	354
243	250	257	264	270	277	284	291	297	304	311	318	324	331	338	345	351	358	365
250	257	264	271	278	285	292	299	306	313	320	327	334	341	348	355	362	369	376
258	265	272	279	286	293	301	308	315	322	329	336	343	351	358	365	372	379	386
265	272	280	287	294	302	309	316	324	331	338	346	353	361	368	375	383	390	397
272	280	287	295	303	310	318	325	333	340	348	355	363	371	378	386	393	401	408
280	288	295	303	311	319	326	334	342	350	358	365	373	381	389	396	404	412	420
287	295	303	311	319	327	335	343	351	359	367	375	383	391	399	407	415	423	431
295	303	312	320	328	336	344	353	361	369	377	385	394	402	410	418	426	435	443

HEALTH STATS

BEFORE THE PROGRAM

Date _____

HRA Score (pages 42–43) _____

Weight _____

BMI _____

Body Fat % _____

Blood Pressure _____

Fasting Cholesterol Total _____

    LDL _____

    HDL _____

    Triglycerides _____

    Cholesterol ÷ HDL Ratio _____

Fasting Glucose _____

AFTER THE PROGRAM

Date _____

HRA Score (pages 42–43) _____

Weight _____

BMI _____

Body Fat % _____

Blood Pressure _____

Fasting Cholesterol Total _____

    LDL _____

    HDL _____

    Triglycerides _____

    Cholesterol ÷ HDL Ratio _____

Fasting Glucose _____

INTERPRETING YOUR HEALTH STATS

Total cholesterol should be less than 200 mg/dl fasting but may be a little higher if not fasting—it is used as a general screen. What matters most is not so much the total cholesterol number but the breakdown of the bad cholesterol (LDL) and good cholesterol (HDL).

LDL cholesterol should be less than 130 mg/dl. In someone with diabetes, the score should be less than 100 mg/dl. In someone with heart disease, the LDL should be less than 70 mg/dl. LDL is usually calculated by an equation that uses the triglycerides score. Because triglycerides are affected by eating, this score will not be accurate unless you have been fasting for twelve hours prior to taking the test.

HDL cholesterol should be greater than 40 mg/dl in men and greater than 50 mg/dl in women. The higher your number is, the lower your risk of heart disease. This score is not affected by eating. Part of what determines this score is genetic, but if you exercise frequently, the score will go up. If you smoke, HDL will rise with smoking cessation.

Triglycerides are affected by what you eat, so the number is best evaluated when fasting. Fasting levels should be less than 150 mg/dl. In insulin resistance (seen in diabetes), the triglyceride level is high and the HDL is low, so sometimes this pattern is an early predictor of diabetes. This number will be greatly reduced by weight loss in those who are overweight and in following guidelines that lower average blood sugar in those who have insulin resistance.

Total cholesterol/HDL ratio should be less than 4.0, preferably less than 3.5; the lower the ratio, the lower the risk for heart disease.

Glucose is affected by how recently you just ate. If you are fasting (no food or drink except water for twelve hours), your score should be less than 100 mg/dl. Your score should never be higher than 140 mg/dl two hours after eating. Fasting scores greater than 125 mg/dl diagnose the condition of diabetes.

HAVE YOU PLEDGED?

Join the millions of Americans taking charge of their health once and for all.

Create one small health pledge you can do over this next year that will help you become healthier and happier. Do you want to eat at least 5 fruits and vegetables a day? Exercise more? Stop smoking?

Think of anything. There is no pledge too small.

Go to

www.healthiestyou.com

When you go to submit your pledge, you will see all of the other health pledges people are entering. You aren't alone. Everyone is trying to get healthier. Join the Movement.

CHANGE YOURSELF.

CHANGE THE NATION.

CHANGE THE WORLD.

ACKNOWLEDGMENTS

THERE ARE MANY PEOPLE who made this book possible. First, I want to thank Robin Straus, my publishing agent, who was able to look at the workbook syllabus I originally presented to her and immediately see what it could become. I also want to thank my coauthor, Betty Sargent, who helped soften my formal medical writing into clear, easy-to-read text. Both have been a delight to work with! I am also grateful to the team at Atria (Simon and Schuster), particularly Johanna Castillo and Judith Curr, who saw the vision for this book right from the start, believed in it, and poured their professional expertise as well as their hearts into it.

I also want to thank my M.D. Health Evolution team: Dean Hovey, Sue Arment, Susan Gilbert, Kurt Atherton, and Kalen Gruber. They supported me, protected my time while writing the book, and shared my hopes that this book could help reach people everywhere to help them succeed in living healthier.

This book would not have been possible without the expertise and hard work of several of my colleagues from Health for Life. Registered dietitians Valerie Koren, Diane Hester, and Laurie Steinberg all contributed to the nutrition content. Physical therapist Merin Powers played a critical role in developing the fitness content. I would also like to thank Marilyn Ferguson-Wolf, Jill Dobson, Stacie Maurer, Patti Caldwell, Marcia Pade, and Elizabeth Schar, for their help in designing the early program model. Getting The Program into an online version was made possible by Jeff Eagle and his team at Eagle Vision. Thank you also to Cathy Heaney, who gave her time and energy for the research study by the Stanford Prevention Research Center in 2007.

A special thank-you goes to the Google Wellness team for supporting this work, particularly Dagan McLennan, who offered unending support and enthusiasm throughout this project and Sue Wuthrich's exceptional vision in employee health. Paul Martini, my illustrator, yet another Google colleague, was amazing in his tireless work to create this book's art. Google physical therapist Mike McTague was also very helpful in rendering his expertise with the fitness illustrations.

I am indebted to all my patients over the years and to all the past and present participants of The Program. You have all served as my teachers and as a source of great inspiration. I also appreciate the endless support of all my amazing friends and colleagues.

Finally, I want to thank my husband, John, and my children, Madeleine, Austin, Tom, Brooke, and Kim, for having the love and patience to help me see this book through completion. My mother, Maureen, and my sisters, Laurie, Kim, and Robin, have also been a wonderful source of strength and support. I'd like to pay a special thank-you to my father, Dean, who we all miss. Thank you for always telling me how much you believed in me, even when I was a small child. It has helped me a lot. Thank you to everyone.

INDEX

ABOUT THE AUTHORS

KELLY TRAVER, M.D., received her medical degree from Stanford, where she also specialized in internal medicine. During an additional year as chief resident, she won the Excellence in Teaching award and currently serves as an adjunct clinical assistant professor of medicine at Stanford. Dr. Traver has been practicing medicine for more than seventeen years, but her background also includes research in biochemistry, teaching in a Stanford neuroanatomy lab, and a brief public health study in South Africa while in medical school. She recently served as medical director at Google and is currently on the board for the Institute for the Future. Dr. Traver is the founder of Healthiest You, a company that works with corporations, health care organizations, and the government to help individuals become more empowered and engaged in their health. She lives with her husband and children in Portola Valley, California.

BETTY KELLY SARGENT is a writer and veteran book and magazine editor, as well as a certified life coach. She is the co-author of *The Instinct Diet* with Susan Roberts, PhD; *Beautiful Bones Without Hormones* with Leon Root, M.D.; and *What Every Daughter Wants Her Mother to Know,* and *What Every Daughter Wants Her Father to Know* with Betsy Perry. She lives in New York City and Tuscany.